Refusing Treatment

This period of 'it ain't gonna change, guv; it's all for the greater good of the NHS'—I'm not sure we'll be here long.

Chief Executive at an NHS trust

Refusing Treatment:
The NHS and market-based reform

Laura Brereton
and
James Gubb

Civitas: Institute for the Study of Civil Society
London

First Published October 2010

ISBN 978-1-906837-19-8

Independence: Civitas: Institute for the Study of Civil Society is a registered educational charity (No. 1085494) and a company limited by guarantee (No. 04023541). Civitas is financed from a variety of private sources to avoid over-reliance on any single or small group of donors.

All publications are independently refereed. All the Institute's publications seek to further its objective of promoting the advancement of learning. The views expressed are those of the authors, not of the Institute.

Typeset by
Civitas

Printed in Great Britain by
Berforts Group Limited
Stevenage SG1 2BH

Contents

	Page
Authors	viii
Acknowledgements	ix
Preface	x
Summary	xi

Refusing Treatment: The NHS and market-based reform

1. Introduction	1
2. Background	5
2.1 Benefits and pitfalls in the use of markets	5
2.2 The switch to a market in the NHS	9
2.3 The way the NHS market operates today	11
2.4 The rationale for introducing a market in the NHS	13
2.5 The productivity imperative facing the NHS	15
2.6 The evidence on the market in the NHS to date	16
3. Methodology	18
3.1 Concepts and scope	18
3.2 Design and sample	19
3.3 Analysis	21
3.4 Limitations	21

Part 1: Is the market working?

4. Core findings	27
4.1 Changes in responsiveness and customer service	27
4.2 No clear impact on equity	30
4.3 Isolated examples of the market driving innovation	30
4.4 Little evidence linking the market to quality improvement	32
4.5 Organisational efficiency up but questionable effects across the system	34
4.6 Discussion	36

Part 2: Why isn't the market delivering greater benefits?

5. Is the concept of a market in the NHS flawed?   41

5.1 The market is considered less effective than other means of
    driving performance in providers   42
    a. Targets, quality initiatives and the open publication of information   42
    b. 'Preferred' providers, PCT self-provision and integrated
      care organisations   43

5.2 Wider problems stemming from markets in health care   45
    a. Collaboration undermined   45
    b. Wasted resources   46
    c. Uninformed and ineffective consumers   47
    d. Profits before patients   48

5.3 Political and centralised nature of the NHS may forever
    quash market incentives   49
    a. Constantly changing policy   50
    b. Government targets   51
    c. Unwillingness to accept hospital closures   52

5.4 Discussion   53
    a. What market?   53
    b. Market mechanisms, even in their current form,
      have still had impact   54
    c. Support for the market structure   55

6. Is the market being distorted and stifled?   57

Part A: Distortions in the market   58

6A.1 Structural imbalance of power between
    purchasers and providers   58
    a. PCTs are too small relative to providers   58
    b. Acute trusts are more established in the health system   59
    c. Practice-based commissioners are underpowered   60

6A.2 Uneven playing field   61

6A.3 Problems with payment-by-results   63

6A.4 The role of GPs   64

6A.5 Discussion   66

Part B: Stifling influences in the market   68

6B.1 Practical obstacles to tendering   69
  a. Lack of alternative options   69
  b. Time consuming tendering processes   71
  c. Bullying from NHS trusts   72
  d. Quality of data questionable   73
  e. PCTs feel locked into relationships with providers   74

6B.2 Underdeveloped skills on the part of purchasers and providers   74
  PCTs   75
    a. Weak management   75
    b. Underdeveloped commissioning skills   76
  Providers   80
    a. 'Classic monopolists'   80
    b. Cost control in NHS providers   81

6B.3 Stifling political and cultural environment   82
  a. Command and control   82
  b. An attachment to the 'comfortable life'   83
  c. Reluctant consumers   84
  d. The 'NHS family'   85

6B.4 Discussion   87

7. What should be done?   90

Annex A: Department of Health guidance on PCT
    procurement and tendering   100

Annex B: Different strategies for procurement and
    contract management   101

Annex C: The NHS in England: The operating framework for
    2008/9 – Principles and rules for co-operation and competition   103

Notes   105

Authors

Laura Brereton holds an MSc in public health/health services management from the London School of Hygiene and Tropical Medicine and a BSc from Boston University (US). She has worked extensively on the impact of ongoing market reforms in the English NHS. Laura is currently a health policy researcher at RAND Europe, where she focuses on health system comparison and chronic disease management. She worked previously in public affairs for health and medical associations in the US and UK.

James Gubb is Director of the Health Unit at Civitas, a post he has held since 2007. His previous publications on health include *Checking up on Doctors: A review of the Quality and Outcomes Framework* and *Putting Patients Last: How the NHS keeps the ten commandments of business failure* (with Peter Davies). James also sits on the steering committee of *Young Civitas for Medics*, a new society set up to involve medical students in health policy discussions, and is a partner in *Streetscape*, a landscape gardening business that strives to take unemployed young people back into work. He is a regular contributor to print, broadcast and healthcare media on issues concerning the NHS.

Acknowledgements

We owe a great debt of gratitude to many people, not least those in the NHS trusts, foundation trusts, PCTs, general practice and private and voluntary sector organisations we selected to study, who volunteered their time to speak to us. For the purposes of this report they remain anonymous, but it is they who made this research possible and we are incredibly grateful.

Also to be mentioned in the same terms are the academics and practitioners who took the time to read, digest and comment on our final draft. Their criticisms and at times brutal honesty have unquestionably enabled us to produce a much more refined report, and we would like to thank them personally.

Finally, we would like to thank our editors, Claire Daley, Anastasia de Waal and David Green, whose input has saved us many errors, inconsistencies and inappropriate turns of phrase. Needless to say, we remain entirely responsible for any that remain.

Preface

As this report entered publication, the new government released a White Paper, *Equity and excellence: Liberating the NHS*, which set out extensive reforms for the NHS. These include dismantling Primary Care Trusts (PCTs), the regional purchasing bodies on whose operation much of this report is focused.

We do not believe this change is necessary to achieve the desired benefits of a functioning market in the NHS, and we are concerned about the implications of further structural change at a time when the NHS faces an unprecedented productivity challenge.

However, the wider commitment to a market in the NHS remains and, as such, the conclusions drawn here on the effectiveness of the PCT-run market for secondary care remain relevant for the NHS, its leaders and researchers, as the NHS enters tight financial times.

While PCTs will be in operation until 2013, the NHS will begin its transformation to a new market structure—one with GP consortia as primary purchasers of care—and our findings may be of interest to those organisations as they begin their own negotiations with acute trusts and other providers. This report's suggestion of separating the Department of Health into purchasing and provision functions has already been put forward in the White Paper, and other recommendations resulting from this work remain highly applicable.

We hope you find this study and its outcomes to be informative and of use as policy initiatives progress.

Laura Brereton and James Gubb
August 2010

Summary

For the past 20 years, the healthcare policies of successive governments have focused to a large extent on developing a market within the NHS in England.

In its latest incarnation (post-2002), the market is administered at the local level by regional purchasers of care, known as Primary Care Trusts (PCTs), and subsidiary groups of GPs, known as practice-based commissioners. Healthcare providers (NHS and non-NHS) compete both for contracts to provide commissioned services, and for individual patients who have free choice of hospital for elective (or planned) procedures.

The reasoning behind the development of this market (from the centrally directed system of purchasing and provision that existed up until the early 1990s) centred primarily on the hypothesis that: if competition, in theory and in practice, has proved to be the greatest single spur to efficiency, quality and innovation in other industries, could it not have the same effect in the NHS?

This report presents the findings of a year-long, in-depth study into whether and why the NHS market has (or has not) driven the perform-ance of healthcare providers as was intended. Based on 46 semi-structured interviews with executives at NHS (foundation) trusts, PCTs, practice-based commissioners and private sector providers across three health economies in England, the study attempts to answer the following questions:

1. Is the market—for contracts with PCTs and, in the case of electives, directly for patients—having its intended impact on the behaviour of secondary care providers?

2. And, if so, is that behaviour bringing about the expected benefits—defined as improved quality, efficiency, innovation, responsiveness to customers, and equity?

The findings are particularly important given the unprecedentedly tight financial times facing the NHS. With a five-year period of near-static real terms increase in funding on the horizon, recent estimates are that, in the face of inflation and rising demand, the NHS will have to obtain in the region of four to six per cent more for its money year-on-year to do little more than maintain existing standards of care.

Core findings

We found isolated examples of the NHS market delivering the benefits that were anticipated; however, the market, by and large, has failed thus far to deliver such benefits on any meaningful or systematic scale. Specifically:

- **Responsiveness to patients has improved**, and acute trusts appear more image-conscious, but the **motivations behind such changes are not clearly linked to the market** in terms of patients having a choice of hospital. Providers tend to be less responsive still to the needs of PCTs as commissioners of care;

- **There has been no clear impact on equity.** There is a risk of inequity in patient choice due to varying, age, socioeconomic status, access to transport and level of education, but this is not supported by hard evidence. However, few PCTs reported using their purchasing power in the market to commission new services targeting those in most need;

- **Isolated examples exist of the market driving innovation.** 'We have clearly indicated... to [consultants] that if we want to compete and retain activity we need to develop new ways of working and new pathways', said one NHS provider executive. However, organisational culture and professional pride were cited more often than market pressure as the motivations behind such actions;

- **Providers gave occasional examples of improvements in quality of care resulting from market pressure, but more often linked such improvements to other factors,** such as the development of an organisation-wide culture of continuous quality improvement; strong local partnerships; a focus on biomedical research; or a desire to achieve high Care Quality Commission (CQC) ratings;

- **Organisational efficiency has improved as a result of the market, but the impact on efficiency across the health system is unclear.** Competitive pressure has incentivised cost-consciousness among acute trusts, and the creation of the post-2002 market coincided with a significant reduction in waiting times. However, although some participants associated this reduction with the (re-) introduction of a market and of Independent Sector Treatment Centres (ISTCs) in particular, others linked it to targets. Participants also cited adverse financial incentives embedded in Payment-by-Results (PbR)—the tariff system for paying secondary care providers—that tends to pull money into acute trusts where it may not be appropriate. One PCT executive remarked '[the market] is bankrupting the system'.

Our analysis led us to consider two possible explanations for why the market has not had the full impact intended:

1. The concept of a market operating in the NHS is flawed and therefore any attempt to introduce one is unlikely to be effective;

2. A market can be effective in the NHS, but it is not currently working because it is being distorted and/or stifled.

Findings in support of the first explanation, that a market can never be truly effective within the NHS, are as follows:

*   Many PCT executives considered that **levers other than the threat of losing business were often more effective in influencing providers**, such as: setting targets; pay-for-performance schemes; peer pressure; and open publication of data;

*   Participants felt the market is **having many of the harmful effects its opponents warned of**, for example, there is evidence that: collaboration is suffering; resources are being wasted; and high quality care is being undermined by organisational self-interest and a 'blame' culture;

*   **Concerns were expressed that market incentives will forever be quashed by the centralised and political nature of the NHS.** The interaction between targets, constantly changing policy, and the demands of the market, led to certain perverse consequences. One provider executive reported: 'right now the contracts and negotiations [with PCTs] are mostly focused on ticking boxes and meeting targets'.

However, there are equally strong problems with the idea that the concept of a market operating within the NHS is flawed:

*   **There is a strong case to be made that such policies have been ineffective because to date there has not been a functioning 'market' in the NHS.** Currently, so many barriers exist to the operation of a market that it seems wrong to draw any concrete

conclusions on its effectiveness.[i] Barriers, for example, have meant that providers are able to operate as monopolies dictating terms to PCTs, rather than competing for PCT business (which has, in fact, produced many of the harmful effects that participants typically attributed to the market);

- Most participants **saw the benefit of the basis of the market; i.e. having a purchasing function (performed by PCTs) separate from providers** that, in the words of one PCT executive, 'represents population and patient interests rather than professional or organisational, and it weighs up clinical opportunities with where the money is spent';

- Examples provided by both commissioners and providers suggest that, although benefits are not currently widespread, **more profound effects would be possible if a market were bedded in**. One PCT executive provided an example: 'We chose to turn to new entrants... and [with these new entrants] there's a vibrancy, a real desire to provide good customer service in a way existing providers were not.'

The alternative explanation as to why the market in the NHS has not delivered the efficiency, quality and innovation expected, is that it is being stifled and distorted. Throughout the course of our study, commissioners and providers reported numerous structural, political, and cultural barriers to the operation of an effective market.

Distortions

- **There is a structural imbalance of power between purchasers (PCTs/practice-based commissioners) and providers (acute trusts).** 'PCTs are scared of the providers' political power', said one provider executive. 'They are afraid of putting services out to

---

[i] In the sample health economy, as of November 2009, only just over half of elective care referrals were made through Choose and Book (a national, computerised, selection system that allows patients to choose their hospital or clinic), meaning nearly half of those referred could not personally choose their provider. Furthermore, the few contracts that had been put out to tender were all small in scope and budget, so even when taken away from existing NHS providers, the contracts had little impact on overall revenue.

tender... and that the hospitals will then go and do something to retaliate that will cause the PCT managers to lose their jobs';

- **There is an uneven playing field between NHS and private/ voluntary sector providers**, resulting in a 14 per cent cost-advantage for NHS providers, when competing for tenders;

- **Payment-by-results for non-elective care creates perverse incentives.** 'If we prevent an admission by good quality care, we lose money', said one provider executive.

Stifling influences

- **A PCT's ability to tender a service, open the market to new entrants, and/or shift services is restricted** by: existing NHS providers operating at 'full' capacity; significant barriers to entry for private and voluntary sector organisations; bullying and predatory pricing by acute trusts; poor data quality; and the bureaucratic and time-consuming nature of the procurement process;

- **PCTs and acute trusts have yet to adapt to operating in a market environment**. In particular, PCT management and commissioning skills—in terms of strategy, decision-making, performance management and tendering—are weak. **Many acute trusts, too, appear either unprepared or ill-equipped to respond to the needs of commissioners**. Cost control is often poor and providers often appear intent on blocking PCT plans;

- **There is a deep cultural reverence for the NHS as something more than a health system.** The emotive notion of the 'NHS family' encourages a counter-productive 'us *versus* them' attitude with regard to the private and voluntary sectors, and has been used in the words of one official 'by most people in most places to try to block [the market]'. We found this to be the most important factor in stifling the market.

On balance we found stronger support for the theory that the NHS market is largely failing to deliver because it is being stifled and distorted than for the theory that it is failing to deliver because its application is fundamentally flawed. While care must forever be taken to preserve the values that the NHS upholds (universal, comprehensive coverage, free-at-the-point-of-use), we strongly encourage the government to support and promote the application of the market as a means out of its financial crisis, and to seek to remove the barriers (not least ministerial influence itself) that are currently distorting and stifling it.

Based on this study, we see the following as a model in which the full potential of the market in the NHS could be achieved:

- There must be a **sustained commitment on behalf of the government to the market** and to principles and parameters that support it. This means:

  o The **Principles and Rules for Cooperation and Competition** as originally formulated in the *NHS Operating Framework 2008/09* (see Annex C) should be re-instated;[1]

  o Consistency in health policy and an end to continuous structural change;

  o That ministers should start telling **a new story for the NHS** as a health service that supports civil society through providing high quality universal, collective, health care coverage, free-at-the-point-of-use, from the best providers available. It should no longer be presented as a culturally revered system of nationalised provision and government focus should be on supporting PCTs as commissioners, not on supporting acute trusts.

- **The Department of Health (DH) should be re-cast from acting as the headquarters of a large corporation of providers to being the 'headquarters' of a commissioning system.** One option for doing so would be to split the DH into provision and commissioning arms:

  o **The provider arm** would be a temporary structure, intended to ensure all secondary care providers that can become foundation trusts do so (regulated by Monitor), and all that cannot are subject to alternative solutions (taken over by other FTs or other independent providers, merged, reconfigured, or where unsustainable, closed);

  o **The commissioning arm (or 'independent commissioning board').** This should *ensure there is an environment conducive to effective commissioning*; develop commissioning skills; define what PCTs are expected to achieve; assess their performance; and institute an appropriate failure regime. Initial tasks should include: developing a more effective and less 'tick-box'-type regulatory framework; encouraging a less burdensome and pre-scriptive approach to tendering; encouraging 'relational' contracting; simplifying standard NHS contracts to shorter forms tailored to contract value; working towards a system of more integrated payment for non-elective care; encouraging PCTs to merge, or work collaboratively, where there is a sound case for doing so; and working towards local contracting of GPs.

- **The role of Strategic health authorities (SHAs)** should be re-cast as out-posts of the 'independent board'.

- **PCTs should be framed along the lines of local health insurers** charged with the goal of securing the best possible health care for their citizens within a constrained budget. They should lose their 'primary/community care' slant and should act as independent, unbiased, evaluators and purchasers for patients free from institutional allegiance (see Chapter 7).

- Providers should be placed in a more **competitive framework**. This would entail:

  o **The Collaboration and Competition Panel (CCP) be given a statutory role** in order to give it real 'teeth' and investigative powers;

  o **Full cost allocation and accounting be enforced.** More specifically, predatory pricing should form part of the remit for the CCP;

  o **Cost disadvantages for the private/voluntary sectors be removed to create a genuinely level playing field.** This applies particularly to pensions;

  o **The publication of comparative data on quality and cost** be advanced, preferably through multiple sources; and regulation should be streamlined across NHS, voluntary and private sector providers;

○ **A proper failure regime for NHS providers, equivalent to going into administration in the private sector, should be instituted,** where assets can be disposed of, taken over or reconfigured according to quality and viability.

We wish to emphasise that we recommend sustaining and supporting the market in the NHS not out of any ideological commitment but based on our findings and those of previous researchers. We see this as the best course of action open to us, as a society, in order to secure high quality care for all in the tight financial times ahead. It will be challenging, but it will also provide an open door to the new ideas and new ways of doing things that the NHS will so desperately need in the coming years.

1

Introduction

The English National Health Service (NHS) is facing what is likely to be its greatest challenge to date. Not only must it cope with a perfect storm of rising expectations, an ageing population, and increasingly expensive medical technology—all of which will increase demand for care—it must do so with the most constrained budget of its 62-year history. Real terms funding[i] for the NHS has never been static or decreased for more than one consecutive year since its foundation in 1948, but the state of the nation's public finances indicates the NHS will almost certainly see at least five consecutive years of near-static real terms growth from 2011/12. The implications are profound: a recent report by The King's Fund and the Institute for Fiscal Studies concludes that in order to do little more than maintain existing standards of care, the NHS will have to achieve productivity gains of four to six per cent per year—equivalent to saving around £40 billion over the coming parliamentary term.[1] And yet maintaining existing standards is unlikely to be accepted by an increasingly consumerist society, who have become accustomed to quicker access to more personalised health services.

Meeting this challenge will not be easy. Despite a 95 per cent real terms increase in funding over the past decade,[2] NHS productivity declined by three per cent between 2001 and 2008 (or 0.4 per cent a year, on average), according to the Office for National Statistics.[3] The single greatest fall of 0.7 per cent occurred in the last year measured, 2008. There is room for improvement in outcomes as well. Although mortality rates from coronary heart disease and cancer have improved,[4] they are still lower than in other OECD countries, as are many standards for the management of chronic diseases.[5]

The question ahead for the NHS must be: how do we secure better health care at lower cost while staying true to the values the NHS embodies: universal, comprehensive health care, free-at-the-point-of-use? Although this is not a new problem, current financial constraints increase the urgency with which we need an answer.

---

[i]   Funding increases after adjusting for economy-wide inflation.

Since 2002—or at least until Gordon Brown became Prime Minister—the solution of the Labour Government was to develop a mixed economy in health care. In essence Labour—consistent with the Conservative Government before them—came to view neither a central regime of targets, nor a simple reliance on the professionalism of doctors, nurses and managers, as the best means to drive performance. Instead, the stimulus for increased quality and efficiency was to be markets and competition. The reasoning was simple: if markets, in theory and in practice, have proved to be the strongest single spur to efficiency, quality and innovation in other industries, could they not have the same effect in the NHS?

The net result of this reasoning is that the NHS is now structured to function on the basis of what has been variously called a 'quasi', 'mimic' or 'internal' market.[6][ii] Central funding is retained but distributed to Primary Care Trusts (PCTs) and groups of GPs known as practice-based commissioners, modelled as impartial agents of patients. PCTs and practice-based commissioners are tasked with buying services from competing secondary and community care providers (NHS and non-NHS) on behalf of their local populations and practice lists. For elective (or planned) procedures, patients have free choice of the hospital to which they are referred. The Department of Health is cast in a supervisory, rather than a direct-managerial, role.

Determining the effectiveness of the NHS market in driving system performance, however, remains something of an elusive pursuit—not least because there is an ongoing debate as to how 'real' the market actually is.[7] Despite an increasing number of academic studies on various aspects of the market, conclusions have tended to be somewhat inconclusive.[iii] Political support for the market structure and related policy appears to be waning, with many asking whether we can afford

---

[ii] For ease of reference, we simply refer to this structure as 'the market' throughout this paper.

[iii] The DH-funded Health Reforms Evaluation Programme, coordinated by Nicholas Mays at the London School of Hygiene and Tropical Medicine, has looked at five aspects of the market reforms and will be reporting in 2010. Other major centres of research in this area include the London School of Economics under Julian Le Grand and The King's Fund.

to take risks with the uncertainties of markets in the tight financial times ahead.

Against this backdrop, we began a 10-month research project with the aim of shedding further light on whether the market in the NHS, as currently configured, is an effective means for improving health system performance. The study was guided by the following core research questions:

a. Is the market—both for contracts with PCTs and, in the case of electives, directly for patients—having its intended impact on the behaviour of secondary care providers?

b. And, if so, is that behaviour bringing about the expected benefits— defined as improved quality, efficiency, innovation, responsiveness to customers, and equity?[iv]

The research was qualitative, consisting of semi-structured interviews with chief executives, finance directors, medical directors, and directors of commissioning at PCTs and practice-based commissioning organisations; NHS trusts; and foundation trusts in one large health economy in England—validated by discussions with executives in two further health economies. In essence, we assemble the thoughts and opinions of people within the different organisations that make up the NHS market and bind them together in an attempt to understand whether the market is working 'on the ground'. We wanted to know how the people whose daily work and decisions drive the market feel about its effectiveness and potential. In doing so, we aspired also to provide insight into *how* and *why* the market is working (or not), in order to highlight future options for policymakers.

This report presents our findings and analysis, along with recommendations for the direction of future policy. It is our hope that the information will be accessible and of interest to the lay reader as well as NHS staff, academics and policy analysts.

The report is structured as follows: Chapter Two explains the contextual background to the research: the history of market reform in the NHS; the economic theory behind the use of markets in healthcare; the productivity imperative facing the NHS; and what is known about

---

iv A full account of our methodology can be found in Chapter 3.

the impact of the market in the NHS to date. Chapter Three describes our methodology. Chapter Four (Part 1) presents core findings—our assessment of the effect the market is currently having against five parameters of success: responsiveness to customers; innovation; quality; equity; and efficiency. Chapters Five and Six (Part 2) are devoted to presenting findings and analysis around why the market is, as yet, failing to deliver anticipated benefits on any meaningful or systematic scale. Our conclusions and policy recommendations are presented in Chapter Seven.

2

Background

There are a number of issues that serve as essential background to understanding the context of the market in the NHS. In this chapter, we review the nature of markets, their benefits and pitfalls, and lessons to take forward in their application to health care. We then look at the historical transition of the NHS to a market-based structure and analyse the processes through which the market is intended to work. We explain the underlying rationale behind the move to a market and the specific benefits that were anticipated, as well as the nature of the productivity imperative now facing the NHS. This chapter concludes by outlining the findings of a literature review[1] carried out in preface to this study and other—more recent—evidence on the effectiveness of the NHS market to date.

2.1. Benefits and pitfalls in the use of markets

Benefits
In the simplest terms, a market is a structure that allows buyers and sellers to exchange a good, service or piece of information. Generally, competitive markets have been shown to deliver better outcomes than monopolistic ones.[2] In competitive markets there tends to be a well developed demand side made up of confident and well-informed consumers, and an efficient supply side made up of different suppliers competing against each other to gain market share.[3][i] Also vital is the ability of new firms with novel, potentially innovative, ideas to enter the market, and the incentive for inefficient firms producing poor quality products or services to exit.[ii] Information is all important. In monopolistic markets, consumers tend to be ill-informed, there are few

---

i   Firms also compete for staff, which gives them powerful incentives to treat their workforce well because staff always have the option of moving elsewhere.

ii   The economist Stephen Nickell has estimated that up to 40 per cent of productivity differences between OECD nations can be accounted for by the level of firm entry and exit. Nickell, S., 'Competition and Corporate Performance', *Journal of Political Economy*, 1996, Vol. 104.

suppliers to choose from, and there is very little entry and exit (if at all). Information tends to be poor. The way competitive markets work is summarised by the Office of Fair Trading and re-produced in Figure 1.[4(iii)]

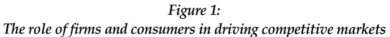

Figure 1:
The role of firms and consumers in driving competitive markets

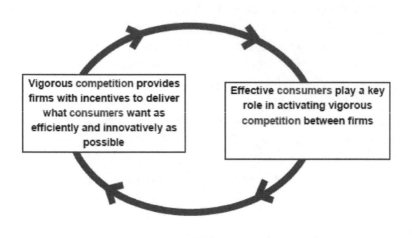

Source: Office of Fair Trading (2010)

However, it is important to realise that markets do not require the 'ideal' (competitive) circumstances described above in order to deliver benefits, for these circumstances frequently do not exist in reality. Typically, to one extent or another there are market failures, such as

---

iii It is worth teasing out the distinction between markets and competition. Competitive markets require competition in the sense that firms are competing for business—typically on the basis of a number of indicators such as price and quality. However, it is possible to have competition without a market (for example, surgeons may compete with each other on the basis of clinical outcomes out of professional pride, without there being any threat of losing business). A market can also exist without much, or any, competition (for example, National Rail before it was privatised).

externalities,[iv] information asymmetry (or uncertainty),[v] and natural monopoly.[5][vi] The success of a market then depends significantly on the effectiveness of regulation and the moral framework in which the market operates.[6] For example:

- Many markets are characterised not by competition between the producers of the goods or services in question, but instead by competition between the suppliers to these producers (such as competition to supply parts to a car manufacturer or diagnostic services to a hospital for an extended period of time). Similar benefits can be seen as in consumer-based markets;[7]

- Markets can and do work in highly regulated industries, such as airlines, telecommunications and eye-care;[8][vii]

- Markets can be used effectively in public services to provide a point of entry for innovative ideas and drive efficiency improvements, even if there is a lack of price signals, a universal service obligation, and a relative absence of profit motive. Local authority tendering is one example.[9]

---

iv An externality is a cost or benefit, not transmitted through prices, that is incurred by a party who did not agree to the action causing the cost or benefit. They can be positive (such as vaccinations) or negative (such as pollution).

v Information asymmetries exist where one party has more or better information than the other. This creates an imbalance of power in transactions which can sometimes cause the transactions to go awry.

vi Natural monopoly arises where the largest supplier in an industry has an overwhelming cost advantage over other actual and potential competitors by virtue of high capital costs (such as public utilities) or of there only being enough consumers to keep one provider in business.

vii The opening of the European aviation market in the 1990s, for example, led to a 66 per cent fall in the lowest (nominal) non-sale fare and a 78 per cent increase in flight frequency between 1992 and 2002. The number of reportable accidents per revenue hour also fell by around 50 per cent. DTI, 'Economics paper no. 9— The Benefits from competition: some illustrative UK cases', 2004, www.berr.gov.uk/files/file13299.pdf (accessed 27 July 2010).

Overall, the benefits of markets can be summarised as follows: they tend to place downward pressure on costs; force firms to focus more on meeting customer needs; lead to more efficient allocations of resources between firms; and act as a spur to innovation and quality improvement.[10] In some circumstances they can also improve equity, by providing choice to those who previously had none.[11] Over the long term, through these means (competitive) markets have generated higher rates of productivity and, in turn, higher economic growth and greater prosperity than any other economic system.[12]

Pitfalls

The problem with markets, however, comes when regulation is poor (as in the recent banking crises) or when the market failures mentioned above—externalities, information asymmetry and natural monopoly— are more pronounced. In such situations, having a market at all may well be inappropriate—the clearest example being policing and law and order. Where markets are deployed in public services, they are unlikely to be effective without 1) significant regulation to protect consumers; and/or 2) government intervention, either to guarantee access or provide services directly.

Health care is a canonical example. As first summarised by Kenneth Arrow, it suffers from a particularly complex combination of market failures: meaningful choice is hobbled due to asymmetries of information between individual users and providers; costs of market entry (financially) and exit (politically and socially) are frequently prohibitive; there is potential abuse of monopoly power; there are interdependencies between consumers' actions (such as a decision to be vaccinated); and there is a large degree of uncertainty over outcomes, meaning price signals do not always work and it is hard to write and enforce contracts.[13] Most importantly, there are also powerful ethical drivers: providers will have other goals than maximisation of profit, and ensuring health care is available to each and every individual regardless of wealth or status is rightly considered a hallmark of a free, fair and just society. We do not expect those who fall seriously ill to have to rely on their bank balance for treatment.

Therefore, if markets are used in health care, there is a difficult balance to strike. Any market must be given the potential to work, and in health care this broadly means: there is an awareness on the part of patients and purchasers (insurers) of the different options available; information on these options can be properly assessed; purchasers (patients and insurers) have the capability to act; there is diversity and flexibility in supply (i.e. entry and exit is possible); and incentives are appropriate.[14] However, any market in health care must also be carefully regulated, with attention forever focused on: preserving universal coverage; the impact on society; and the potential consequences of market failure. Careful consideration must also be given to the processes through which competition is encouraged;[viii] the type and quality of information that is made available to patients (which often determines the indicators on which providers will compete); and the ways in which providers/insurers are remunerated.[15][ix] Using a market may also be inappropriate for certain services where there are natural monopolies, such as the provision of specialist neurology.

2.2. The switch to a market in the NHS

Throughout its history, the NHS has not typically functioned as a market. In fact, NHS providers have mostly enjoyed operating with monopoly status. Despite numerous structural reorganisations, the Secretary of State for Health and the Department of Health (DH) traditionally supervised regional and sub-regional health authorities directly, with regional health authorities holding devolved budgets and directly managing hospital and community health services.

This changed when the Conservative Government's 1989 White Paper *Working for Patients* was enshrined in the 1990 NHS and Community Care Act. The key tenet of the paper's reforms was to separate organisations into the roles of purchaser and provider.[16] District health authorities (DHAs) were dissolved of their responsibility

---

viii For example, should patients have choice of secondary care provider at the point of referral, choice of general practice, or choice of health insurer; or should competition mainly be in the form of hospitals bidding for service contracts with insurers/government agencies?

ix Different types of remuneration may be appropriate for different services. For example, it may be appropriate to pay by activity in elective care if the intention is to increase activity and thereby reduce waiting times, but paying by activity is unlikely to be appropriate for the management of long-term conditions, where a goal may be to encourage self-care.

for directly managing hospitals and instead were given per capita, weighted budgets to purchase health services from newly formed healthcare trusts and other organisations. Groups of GP 'fundholders' (primary care physicians), could also choose to take on budgets to buy a subset of elective (planned) care for their patients. NHS healthcare trusts were then expected to compete to offer the best services in terms of cost, quality and convenience. For the first time, a market was introduced to the NHS.

Upon coming to power in 1997, the Labour Government initially sought to draw back on the idea of a market in favour of 'collaboration' and 'partnership', although the purchaser/provider split was maintained. In practice, however, the years 1997-2002 are perhaps best described as a centralised regime of 'targets and terror',[17] where heavy emphasis was placed on driving performance through what has been termed 'hierarchical challenge'.[18]

In 2002 the tide changed again, back to an emphasis on markets and competition—only this time Labour went further than their Conservative predecessors. On the demand side of the market, Primary Care Trusts (PCTs)—the latest incarnation of DHAs—were handed the legal duty to 'secure the best services, in terms of quality and productivity, for the people they serve', be it from NHS, private or voluntary sector providers.[19] Such commissioning (or procurement) was to be carried out through a process of 'assessing local health needs, identifying the services required to meet those needs and then buying those services from a wide range of healthcare providers'.[20] GP fundholding, too, was re-instated in the form of 'practice-based commissioning' (PbC), though this time with virtual, rather than real, budgets and focused on the management of long-term conditions and community services, rather than on elective procedures. Within electives, patients were instead given the right to choose between 'any willing provider' meeting DH standards and prices—including from the private and voluntary sectors—through a new national, computerised, selection system called Choose and Book.

Reforms were also made on the supply side. NHS trusts (the healthcare trusts established through the 1990 reforms) that met certain standards of finance, quality and governance were encouraged to apply for additional independence through becoming foundation trusts

(FTs).[x] In order to further stimulate competition between providers, centrally-negotiated contracts were offered to private sector organisations from around the globe to set up treatment centres in England to carry out elective and diagnostic procedures on behalf of the NHS. These clinics became known as Independent Sector Treatment Centres (ISTCs).

To complete the reform package, new rules and regulations were introduced to support the market. For the majority of procedures, secondary care providers no longer receive payment through lump-sum annual block contracts, but per case at a (now maximum) tariff set by the DH, adjusted for case mix, a market forces factor[xi] and—since 2009—incentive payments for quality (CQUIN[xii]). Income is thus dependent on a provider's ability to attract business and on the quality of care offered. On top of this, regulators have been introduced to help guarantee financial viability (Monitor, for foundation trusts), quality of care (the Care Quality Commission) and quality of commissioning (the DH's 'World Class Commissioning' assurance regime, introduced in 2008). More recently (2008/09) rules around procurement, tendering and competition (including entry and exit) have been introduced, which form the terms of reference for the NHS Competition and Collaboration Panel (CCP).

2.3 The way the NHS market operates today

In many ways the market that emerged in the NHS under the Labour Government exemplifies the balancing of structures and incentives necessary to garner benefits from the market, with the need to preserve universal coverage and protect against market failure (see section 2.1). Two things in particular should be noted. The first thing is the

---

[x]   FTs are public benefit corporations able to take on a range of extra freedoms, such as the ability to retain profits for investment and access private capital.

[xi]   Market forces factor (MFF) is a way of adjusting allocations to purchasers for unavoidable geographical variations in healthcare costs. MFF takes into consideration cost variations in land, buildings, equipment and staff pay (including a London weighting).

[xii]   Commissioning for Quality and Innovation.

processes through which the current market works (or is intended to work). In essence, there are two:

a. Providers competing for contracts with PCTs (or their subsidiaries, practice-based commissioners) to provide particular services, through a process of competitive tendering;[xiii]

b. Providers competing for individual patients who, for purposes of elective care, can choose where they wish to receive treatment.[21]

Prices are currently fixed by the payment-by-results tariff for most secondary care procedures (including electives), and providers are paid per case. However, prices are variable when it comes to bidding for contracts outside the remit of the tariff, such as community services, mental health care and general practice. It is important to emphasise, too, that market activity is primarily focused on secondary care. There is little by way of a market for general practice, although tenders have been issued for *new* services and there are moves to introduce a more formalised choice of general practice for patients (i.e. outside current geographic boundaries); and there is little specific attention given to developing a market around the management of chronic conditions. Also important is that there is no choice of 'commissioner', rather PCTs and practice-based commissioners enjoy geographic monopolies.

The second thing to note is market incentives are far from the only incentives facing organisations in the NHS. Particularly because the NHS remains a single-payer health system, funded through general taxation, the government retains considerable influence over the terms of play and has, over the past ten years, used this to set targets that organisations are expected to meet (the Care Quality Commission, for example, currently assesses organisations against 69 national targets set by government, largely relating to waiting times and processes of care). From 2009, secondary care organisations can also lose income under the CQUIN scheme if they do not meet certain quality indicators (as general practice does under the Quality and Outcomes Framework). Additionally, provider organisations will be concerned with satisfying a number of other constituencies: regulators; strong trade unions; local

---

[xiii] There are also sub-markets emerging through NHS (foundation) trusts contracting certain services out to private and voluntary sector providers.

politicians; patient groups; and the local media, to name but a few. They also have strong ethical drivers, deriving from the caring, collaborative nature of medicine and the professionalism of the staff they employ.

2.4 The rationale for introducing a market in the NHS

If one word could be used to describe the underlying motivation behind the 2002 market-based reforms, it would be 'frustration': frustration that the billions of pounds being pumped into the NHS were not bringing the desired results (most particularly, falls in waiting times), and frustration that ministerial direction seemed unable to do much about it. In essence, Labour—consistent with the Conservative Government before them—came to view neither a central regime of 'targets and terror', nor a simple reliance on the professionalism of doctors, nurses and managers, as sufficient means to drive performance in the NHS. The language used in the 2002 White Paper, *Delivering the NHS Plan,* is indicative:

> The 1948 model [for running the NHS] is simply inadequate for today's needs. We are on a journey... that represents nothing less than the replacement of an outdated system. We believe it is time to move beyond the 1940s monolithic top-down centralised NHS towards a devolved health service, offering wider choice and greater diversity bound together by common standards, tough inspection and NHS values.[22(xiv)]

The aim, as laid out more explicitly in a 2005 paper published by the DH, was to achieve a 'self-improving' NHS with an 'inbuilt dynamic for

---

xiv The document went on to list a catalogue of 'profound and historical weaknesses' in the NHS: chronic capacity shortages; weak or perverse incentives that inhibit performance; an absence of explicit patient choice; lack of co-operation between public and private provision exacerbated by separate regulatory systems; a top-down, centralised system that inhibits local innovation; health and social care systems that work against each other when older people particularly need them to work together; out-dated working practices which have prevented a more rational design of services and deployment of staff; lack of attention to the rights and responsibilities of patients; and weak local and national accountability.

continuous improvement... not designed as a blueprint for *how* services should be delivered [but as] a means to improvement', i.e. a market.[23(xv)]

The arguments put forward for introducing such a market were in essence the same as those put forward in support of markets more generally (and in relation to public services) explained in section 2.1. First, introducing a market was seen as an important way of promoting competition between providers—both for patients in the case of electives and for contracts from PCTs in the case of other services—thus sharpening incentives to be efficient and increasing capacity in the hospital sector where differences in waiting times existed. Second, in introducing a market, the government aimed to encourage providers to be more responsive to patients' (and commissioners') preferences and to drive improvements in quality. An increase in innovation was also anticipated, the idea being that when either patients or commissioners leave (or threaten to leave) a low-quality provider, the provider would notice and use it as an impetus either to improve quality to stay in the market, or to exit from the market. Similarly, high quality providers would have the incentive to become even better in order to gain more custom.[24]

That said, to couch the anticipated benefits of the NHS market purely in economic terms is wrong; social benefits were also anticipated. In engineering an NHS that embraced choice, quality and responsiveness for all, without charges or selection by wealth, Labour also hoped to enhance equity. As the then Prime Minister Tony Blair said in 2003:

> Choice mechanisms enhance equity by exerting pressure on low-quality or incompetent providers. Competitive pressures and incentives drive up quality, efficiency and responsiveness in the public sector. Choice leads to higher standards. The overriding principle is clear. We should give poorer patients... the same range of choices the rich have always enjoyed. In a heterogeneous society, where there is enormous variation in needs and preferences, public services must be equipped to respond.[25]

[xv]   The most clear-cut notion of this came with the ISTC programme, which carried the explicit aim of 'spread[ing] new ways of working, spur[ring] NHS providers to increase their responsiveness to patients and, as a result of increased contestability, driv[ing] down the level of inefficient spot purchasing'.
Department of Health, *NHS Improvement Plan: Putting People at the Heart of Public Services*, London: TSO, 2004.

In embracing such a model, Labour held the additional aim of building greater solidarity around the NHS's core values, among rich and poor alike.[26] In 2004, Blair said: 'we are completely re-casting the 1945 welfare state to end entirely the era of "one size fits all" services... [to] ensure that we keep our public services universal, for the middle classes as well as those on low income'.[27]

2.5 The productivity imperative facing the NHS

It should be recognised that the political and economic environment in which the market in the NHS was (re-)introduced in the early-to-mid 2000s is very different to that facing the NHS now. Between 1999/2000 and 2009/10, real terms funding for the NHS increased by 95 per cent.[28] However, the current state of the nation's public finances means an unprecedented five-year period of near-static real terms increase in funding is now on the horizon. The King's Fund and Institute for Fiscal Studies recently analysed the implications of this for the NHS, by setting scenarios for real terms funding against that projected as necessary to meet demand by Sir Derek Wanless for HM Treasury in 2002.[29] With the NHS now closer to the least optimistic of Wanless's projections (having seen falling productivity and poor population engagement in health), the shortfalls envisaged can be seen in Table 1 (p. 16)

The Coalition Government has committed to real term increases in funding for the NHS over the course of the next parliament. However, the impact on funding for other government departments means this is likely to be near zero, leaving the NHS with an estimated funding gap of approaching £40bn by 2015/16, requiring *annual* productivity improvements in the order of four to six per cent. It is worth emphasising what this means: after the NHS has achieved four to six per cent more output per unit of input in the first year, it will have to do the same in the second year, dealing with inputs that are already four to six per cent leaner than the first; the same in the third year with inputs that are some four to six per cent leaner again and so on until the fifth year. To provide an indication of this difficulty, average productivity across UK private sector industry increased by 2.3 per cent per annum over the past decade;[30] some two to four per cent less than that now required in the NHS. New service models are likely to be essential.

Table 1:
The NHS's productivity imperative

Year/period	Annual productivity gains required to fill funding gap with Wanless's least optimistic scenario (slow uptake)					
	Average annual change (%)			Total for period (£m, 2010/11 prices)		
	Artic[xvi]	Cold[xvii]	Tepid[xviii]	Artic	Cold	Tepid
2011/13	8.2	6.2	4.2	26,033	19,683	13,334
2014/16	6.8	5.8	2.8	21,429	18,255	8,730
Whole period	7.5	6.0	3.5	47,462	37,938	22,064

Source: The King's Fund/IFS (2009)

2.6 The evidence on the market in the NHS to date

One hope is that the market in the NHS will help to drive such productivity improvements. However, there are reasons to doubt this and, more widely, to doubt whether the market can deliver the anticipated benefits described in section 2.3—efficiency, quality, innovation, responsiveness and equity.

As highlighted in section 2.1, health care does not lend itself naturally to market-based provision due to a number of market failures, not least asymmetry of information and uncertainty. Health care markets also tend to be quite heavily concentrated (i.e. monopolistic).[31] Looking at the wider literature, evidence on the effectiveness of markets in health care is inconclusive. To take one example, studies on

---

xvi Annual real reductions of two per cent for the first three years, falling to one per cent for the final three years.

xvii Zero real change in funding across the six years.

xviii Annual real increases of two per cent for the first three years, increasing to three per cent for the final three years.

markets for hospital care have found a significant and positive relationship between market concentration (a proxy for the level of competition) and higher quality, on indicators such as mortality rates, patient satisfaction and patient safety, where prices are regulated. However, where prices are variable, the outcome is mixed, with studies highlighting negative as well as positive consequences.[32] In 2006, Carol Propper and colleagues concluded that 'there is neither strong theoretical nor empirical support for competition', while noting that there are cases where competition has led to improved outcomes.[33]

The picture is also unclear when looking specifically at the market in the NHS. The most recent research shows the market having notable, positive effects. In particular, studies indicate that, where competitive, the market has tended to: improve managerial quality; reduce inequalities in access (in terms of waiting times); improve quality as measured by 30-day in-hospital mortality from acute myocardial infarction; and reduce length-of-stay, while controlling costs.[34] All are significant findings. However, a review of the literature in early 2010 suggests that while the market has contributed to improved access for patients, reduced waiting times and increased efficiency in providers, the breadth of benefits is not yet close to that seen in other sectors— particularly with regard to innovation.[35] In particular, market incentives appear to be weakened and mangled by a policy environment that is in a constant state of change, with the basic diffusion of information on quality and cost that markets rely on remaining suboptimal. The impact of the market on the social fabric of the NHS also remains unclear, with media and political commentators drawing attention to the danger bringing markets into the NHS presents in terms of trust, social citizenship, solidarity and equality.[36] There is a very lively debate, led by the British Medical Association and other trade unions, on whether or not the market should be abandoned completely.[37] It is against this backdrop that the importance of this study is cast.

3

Methodology

3.1 Concepts and scope

As stated, the broad aim of our study was to shed light on whether the market in the NHS, as currently configured, is an effective means for driving the performance of providers, and in turn, whether it is bringing benefit to patients, staff and the system as a whole.

From this, we worked to refine the focus to something we could reasonably answer with a 10-month study. Background research and scoping included a large-scale literature review of existing evidence on the impacts of market policy in the NHS to date;[1] a review of market theory and its application to health care;[2] and a review of the literature on quality in health care (unpublished). We also spoke with many academic healthcare researchers, and past and present NHS executives. Ultimately, we arrived at the following core research questions:

a. Is the market—for contracts with PCTs and, in the case of electives, directly for patients—having its intended impact on the behaviour of secondary care providers?[i]

b. And, if so, is that behaviour bringing about the expected benefits—defined as improved quality, efficiency, innovation, responsiveness to customers, and equity?[ii]

In answering these questions we also aimed to provide insight into *how* and *why* the market is (or is not) working in order to illustrate future policy options. We chose to focus on secondary care providers because this is where the market in the NHS is most established and where the majority of market-based policy over the past decade has been targeted. In referring to the NHS market, we mean the structures

---

i By secondary care providers we mean any provider of acute services for which patients typically require a GP referral to access.

ii This definition derives from a search of available literature on quality in health care, and from an analysis of government documents highlighting the benefits anticipated, as outlined in section 2.3.

and policies that allow commissioners (PCTs and practice-based commissioners) to buy services from providers and that allow patients to choose between providers (in the case of elective care)—the structures, in other words, that present the specific threat and opportunity to providers of gaining and losing business.

3.2 Design and sample

We opted for a qualitative research methodology primarily because we wanted to not only provide insight into *whether* the market appears to be working, but also *how* and *why* it is (or is not) working. We wanted to understand the impact the market is having on what people and organisations are doing (and not doing), why they are (or are not) doing it, and what impacts these actions are having on patients and on society.

With this in mind, we decided to run the study as a series of semi-structured interviews with people who are effectively determining the success of the NHS market through their day-to-day work and decisions. The semi-structured nature enabled us to maintain reliability of questioning while allowing participants to expand on related issues and add personal insight.

Lines of questioning focused on a number of topics including: the participant's role and view of his/her organisation; recent experiences; the motivation behind various decisions, such as developing services and tendering; and opinions of the impact of current market structure and policies on each. The questions were developed and tested through pilot interviews with organisations not directly involved in the study. Participants were also given the opportunity to speak about the market directly and were allowed to introduce issues we may not otherwise have come across. The time period examined was post-2002, and our focus was on the NHS in England, as the degree to which market forces have been used in health care differs within the other countries that make up the United Kingdom.

The interview sample we adopted was drawn purposefully. Given that in theory and practice, markets—in regulated industries—are likely to be most effective in areas of low concentration,[3][iii] we chose to focus the study on a large conurbation with a comparatively low Herfindahl-Hirschman Index (HHI)[iv] and where no single acute trust could be seen as the dominant provider in terms of the market share of services commissioned by local PCTs.[v] We hypothesised that market concentration would be one of the most relevant and objective circumstances to the phenomenon being studied:[4] the success, or otherwise, of the market in such a geographic area will have important implications for the success of such policies in areas without such a supportive attribute.[vi]

Within this health economy, our sample consisted of five NHS trusts (of which three are foundation trusts); three PCTs; an ISTC; practice-based commissioners; an area-wide collaboration of PCTs; and a number of private providers that had entered the market in recent years, seeking to take advantage of the patient choice initiative. We interviewed three executives and a lead consultant at each NHS (and foundation) trust; three executives at each PCT; PbC group representatives; two executives at one of the local private providers; and a number of other academic and political informants. In the few cases where the chosen person was unable to participate, a deputy or close colleague was interviewed instead. In total, 46 interviews were

---

iii   Concentration is a function of the number of producers (in this case, healthcare providers) and their respective shares of total production (health service provision). The lower the market concentration, the more providers there are in an area and the less it resembles a monopoly — therefore, the greater the potential for competition.

iv   Data provided by Carol Propper of Imperial College, University of London. The HHI is a measure of the size of firms in relation to the industry and an indicator of the amount of competition among them. It can range from 0 to 1.0, moving from a large number of very small firms to a single monopolistic producer. Increases in the HHI generally indicate a decrease in competition and an increase of market power, whereas decreases indicate the opposite.

v   Proprietary data maps provided by PA Consulting.

vi   We could have chosen to spread time and resources across more than one geographic area, but we felt it would be more fruitful to strive for a deeper understanding of how the market is functioning in one region (rather than obtaining surface level impressions of many).

carried out between October and December 2009. Interviews were predominantly in-person, lasting around 30 minutes, and followed the basic topic structure outlined above.

Because of past experience suggesting that tape recorders can inhibit participants from expressing their true feelings, interviews were transcribed by hand, typed immediately afterwards, and sent back to interviewees to check and amend. Only the changed, confirmed versions were used in analysis. Consent and anonymity was considered an ongoing process. For this reason, we do not refer to our sample location by name, nor do we mention names of individual organisations, people, or job titles in quote attribution in this report.

3.3 Analysis

Following the conclusion of the interview stage, all interview transcripts were reviewed individually by two researchers. Paying particular attention to any impacts that could be linked to the market (relating to our five parameters of success: responsiveness and customer service; quality of care; efficiency; equity; and innovation), we noted repeated phrases or sentiments, as well as any outlying responses. Before being written up, all coded data, including direct quotations, were transferred to separate, themed documents and categorised by response of purchaser or provider.

We sought to validate our findings by discussing the results with two acute trusts and PCTs in two separate areas in England, one metropolitan and one more rural. This was helpful in allowing us to hear how their experiences compared with what we had found, and informed us of the extent to which we might be able to generalise the results. Where interviewee opinions differ, they are explained.

3.4 Limitations

As with any study design, there are limitations to the approach we have taken, which readers should bear in mind throughout:

1. Qualitative work alone cannot fully answer the question: 'Is the market working?'; respondents can give their *view* on whether the organisation they work for is becoming more efficient, for example, but a quantitative study would be needed to ascertain that the

organisation *has* in fact become more efficient. Rather, the value of qualitative work—relating to the questions we have posed—lies in providing a ground-level *impression* of how effective the market has been, and, perhaps even more so, in providing insight into *how* and *why* the market is working (or not).

2. There are difficulties in attributing specific outcomes to a single (and multi-faceted) variable—in this case, market reforms. The two-step question we have employed, looking first at changing behaviours and then the benefits that may be derived from the market, attempts to address this issue; but the complexity of the NHS's structure, frequent policy change (such as the change of emphasis from markets to pay-for-performance following Lord Darzi's review of the NHS in 2008), funding increases and wider social trends present multiple confounding factors.

3. Response bias is another concern with qualitative interviews.[vii] We attempted to address this by piloting our interview questions and discussing them with academic informants to try to remove any potential leads in questioning.

4. Because of the limited time and resources available, coupled with our desire to speak with those whose day-to-day decisions most impact the functioning of the market, the majority of interviewees were in high-level managerial positions. Whilst this included medical directors and clinical leaders, we would like to have obtained more 'frontline' clinical input.

5. A key challenge for us has been determining the external validity (or 'generalisability') of our results, given that they are based predominantly on one health economy and could very well say more about experiences and relationships in this area than about the impact of the NHS market across England. This is a concern, but we believe our findings can sufficiently support the conclusions we draw due to: i) our selection of a sample area conducive to the success of a market (and the implications we can knowingly draw

---

vii This, for example, includes the tendency for people to present a favourable image of themselves or their organisation; or answer questions along the lines he/she thinks the interviewer desires.

elsewhere), and ii) validation interviews carried out in two other health economies so that idiosyncrasies could be identified and further analysed.

Our contribution to the debate is to provide in-depth insight into how the NHS market is operating 'on the ground', to assemble the thoughts and opinions of people across the different organisations that make up the NHS market, and to bind them together in an attempt to assess how effective the market has been, and why.

PART 1: Is the market working?

4

Core findings

The direct answer to our first research question, 'Is the market—for contracts with PCTs and, in the case of electives, directly for patients— having its intended impact on the behaviour of secondary care providers?', is, at best, 'a little'. The answer to our second question, 'If so, is that behaviour bringing about the expected benefits—defined as improved quality, efficiency, innovation, responsiveness to customers, and equity?' is closer to 'no', except in isolated instances. By and large we did not find the market as it is currently operating—defined either by patient choice or by PCT tendering—to have been an especially powerful catalyst in driving the behaviour of secondary care providers. And, where we did see it having an effect on actions and decisions, rarely was there a clear link to the improvements in patient care that were envisaged. These findings were evident both in our sample health economy and in the two geographical areas we selected as part of our validation process. As one provider executive put it, 'I don't think it [the market] is working as intended.'

Before entering into a more extensive analysis as to why this may be so, this chapter is devoted to reviewing the specific impact, or lack of impact, we found the market to be having on the behaviour of providers in association with each parameter of anticipated benefit— improved quality; efficiency; innovation; responsiveness to customers; and equity—and discussing the implications of these findings.

4.1 Changes in responsiveness and customer service

Responsiveness to patients
Overall, the majority of provider executives we interviewed felt under increased pressure to ensure their organisation treated patients as 'people' and 'customers'. As one executive put it:

> NHS staff don't like the word 'customer'... the NHS has always dealt with vulnerable people. But I have seen a growing emphasis on promoting the little things, for example, are staff approaching people who look lost in the corridors?

However, the extent to which this permeated the focus of leadership agendas varied. Disagreement also existed on the source of this pressure to be more 'customer-orientated', with interviewees attributing it to many things including organisational pride; external pushes from the DH; 'market-based policies'; and a new sense of freedom associated with FT status. 'Interestingly, people, particularly medical staff, behave differently when they perceive themselves to be free of central control and can make a difference', said one chief executive. 'It's a psychological issue.'

The introduction of patient choice itself did not appear to stimulate providers to be more responsive to patients' desires as consumers, quite possibly because providers are currently not seeing any great effect from the policy. Not one provider executive reported patient choice to have had a significant impact on patient numbers ('we've not seen any impact...' was a typical response); nor did they express a particular concern for losing patients ('for most patients, choice [to go elsewhere] is low on their agenda'). Neither did the existence of a nearby ISTC appear to have had much effect on the decisions or business strategies of providers in our sample health economy. As one executive at a private provider said:

> You would have thought that if the ISTC is doing business, NHS trusts are missing out on it, but they've not been very vocal about this.

Most providers we spoke to—including in our validation sites—did not feel compelled to make changes in order to attract patients.

That said, subtle impacts of choice policy were noted. In particular, providers appeared acutely image-conscious. One executive outlined how:

> We are trying to change the image we project. We are spending some capital revamping the front of the hospital, for example. At the moment it looks very domestic and higgledy-piggledy.

Others mentioned actively marketing services to patients and GPs: 'we try to get the message out [that] we have lower MRSA, *C-diff* and waiting times than other trusts', said one. Another participant felt that a nearby FT's advertising had helped it to pull in a small proportion of patients from 'border areas' (where the FT and another NHS trust were equidistant). This was confirmed by executives at the FT, who felt their large speciality diagnostic and treatment centres played a role in attracting non-local patients as well as commissioned services.

Responsiveness to PCTs as commissioners of care

One would expect that PCTs, holding the 'purse strings' of the NHS at a local level and having the power to move services elsewhere in the light of poor performance, would command significant influence over providers. However, this was not the impression we obtained. In fact, executives at both PCTs and providers agreed that for the most part providers held the power in their relationships. As one PCT executive put it:

> Unlike other PCTs [in the region], we spend only about 35 per cent on our largest provider—our purchasing is diversified, so theoretically we stand to gain from NHS market policy. So far this has not happened.

Another explained:

> Providers have more negotiating power because they are bigger... the consultants are right there involved in decisions... [and they] have the patients on their side. Everyone loves their local hospital.

Indeed, for many provider executives, whether or not PCTs would pay for a service expansion appeared to be almost an after-thought.

However, in certain circumstances PCTs did report minor changes in provider responsiveness when services had been put out to tender. One PCT executive explained:

> [We are more able to positively influence providers] on services we have recently commissioned than those that have been contracted for a while. Often [in older contracts] the structures just are not in place to measure and manage provider performance. It is a reason to go through a rigorous procurement process and ask potential providers how they foresee us working together to make changes and improvements.

In particular, PCTs—and especially those in our validation sites— gave evidence of an increased willingness on the part of providers in new contracts to negotiate and update contracts, or to offer service changes desired by the PCT. The ongoing problem, however, was that existing NHS providers, at least in our sample health economy, often resorted to threats (explicit or implied) and/or expensive and time-consuming legal action if a tender resulted in a change of provider.

29

4.2 No clear impact on equity

Participants in our sample health economy expressed the concern that patient choice may work to the detriment of people from lower socioeconomic groups. One PCT executive put it as such:

> The market right now is contested on the basis of economic mobility. People who have access to the internet and who are educated enough to be able to know where to look, can find the best providers and ask to be referred to them. Patient choice is currently inequitable in terms of age, socioeconomic status, and level of education.

While this comment is anecdotal, an analysis we carried out of the patient profile at a nearby ISTC does suggest it is the middle-classes who are predominantly choosing to go there (but not that the ISTC is 'cherry-picking' them). Another participant noted that aside from education, for many patients, an obvious obstacle to choice is poor access to transport.

Looking outside the domain of patient choice, the wider question is whether PCTs have been able to use their purchasing power in the market to commission services that are more appropriate for disadvantaged groups than the traditional settings of the hospital and general practice. We saw little evidence of this other than the commissioning of new sexual health and dentistry services. As one PCT executive described:

> There is certainly a huge amount of unmet need, but [at present] the 'savvy consumers' tend to be the ones who get the treatment. What we are not doing is improving access and detection of need.

4.3 Isolated examples of the market driving innovation

The potential for the market—in terms of competition for both PCT contracts and elective patients—to stimulate innovation in the NHS was widely acknowledged by participants at both purchaser and provider organisations. As one provider executive put it:

> It makes you start to think about what you need/want to do for patients, what is possible, rather than just continuing with what you are familiar with.

Some PCT executives were able to provide examples of where this had happened in practice. As one explained:

[A regional, independently run, one-stop diagnostic centre] had an unexpected, positive impact on the actions and priorities of local acute trusts... such as reconfiguring their outpatient services to do the same... it is the view of some that this wouldn't have happened otherwise.

Many, too, felt that the threat of competition, perhaps more than competition itself, could act as motivation for providers to look at new ways of delivering services. One PCT executive said:

The idea of competition and the existence of independent providers has stimulated innovation in some cases, providing incentives for NHS providers to make changes.

Participants in the validation interviews outside our sample health economy provided concrete examples, such as the introduction of a new community diabetic service forcing hospitals to focus on having fewer follow-up appointments; and a PCT tender motivating the introduction of a new physiotherapy-led triage system that enables orthopaedic surgeons to see patients more appropriate for surgery, maximising their operating time.

We were also told that providers had actively used the 'threat'— whether real or otherwise—from PCTs that they would purchase services elsewhere as a positive impetus. One provider executive reported:

We have actually used the threat of competition as a lever for internal change here, particularly regarding service innovation. We have shown consultants the gaps in their practice and clearly indicated to them that if we want to compete and retain activity, we need to develop new ways of working and new pathways.

A more profound impact was seen in another acute trust. One executive said:

We are surrounded by organisations that have outflanked us... They have been more ambitious in making bids for services and expanding, and have shown more flexibility in expanding to meet demand. [We have] achieved the remarkable feat of missing the gravy train.

Another executive at the same trust reported:

Our strategy [now] revolves around finding a unique selling point in this market that allows us to survive and provide services locally. We are thus looking at new models of care to take out hospital beds and developing primary care services with GPs to manage long-term conditions in people's homes.

31

That said, only a minority of participants were able to provide evidence of innovation coming about as a direct result of competitive pressure, suggesting that overall impact has been limited. 'I haven't felt any great shift I would connect with [the market]', remarked one PCT executive in reference to any impact of the market on innovation. Others contradicted the aforementioned view that the introduction of independent providers through the centrally-negotiated ISTC programme had had any significant effect. As one executive put it:

> I've not really seen any impact... the interface is poor; tests are often repeated. And [the independent sector] can 'cherry-pick' easier cases.[i]

PCT executives also expressed frustration that the immediate response of NHS providers tended to be protectionist, rather than responsive, thereby annulling any potential for innovation deriving from the market. In reaction to an independent provider being brought in to our sample health economy, for example, NHS acute providers immediately formed a cartel and refused to let their consultants work with, or at, the new clinic. Perhaps illuminating the overall situation, few provider executives mentioned competition as a significant driver for change; most cited targets, CQC ratings (quality of services/use of resources), local patient need, professional pride and wider regional/ SHA plans as their primary motivation in making service changes.

4.4 Little evidence linking the market to quality improvement

Similar to findings on innovation, few provider executives made any direct link between the market and quality improvement. Instead, most attributed successes to other factors, such as the development of an organisation-wide culture of continuous quality improvement, strong local partnerships, and a focus on biomedical research. One provider executive reported:

> Competition has not been our driving force. Our organising principles have been centred on quality and safety, which has attracted partners.

---

[i]   This was a specific reference to ISTCs. However the extent to which ISTCs 'cherry-pick' patients can be disputed because it is in their contracts to provide particular procedures for particular groups of patients (i.e. those without complex co-morbidities).

Motivations for quality improvement were more often tied to information published on performance than to a need to compete for either contracts or patients. As one provider executive put it:

> My opening approach to trust strategy was driven by the question: How do we get to 'good/good' CQC ratings? We don't want to be the only trust in [the region] without 'good/good' ratings.

However, many did associate increased independence, particularly foundation trust status, with quality improvement. As one PCT executive said:

> The need for trusts to become or stay financially independent has helped to drive quality, probably more so than block contracts [which went before].

A few provider executives also reported using the market environment as a tool to drive performance—whether or not they felt the threat of losing 'business' was genuine. One provider executive reported:

> There is pressure to compete for patients and [an] awareness that money follows patients. I would hope that it affects care in a positive way—improving quality and waiting times in order to attract referrals. I have seen this work as a motivator here, and with recruitment as well; we want to attract the sort of clinicians who want to move services forward.

PCTs, too, generally considered the ability to turn to alternative providers to be a useful lever, when used appropriately. As one executive detailed:

> We have certainly brought in new providers as a deliberate move to improve performance [in areas such as dentistry and sexual health] and I believe this has worked as an incentive for others to increase quality.

With regard to quality in newer, non-NHS providers, however, opinions were mixed. Some executives were highly complimentary. 'I can't fault the care at [the ISTC]. Clinically, it's superb', said one medically-qualified executive. Another said, in reference to the same provider: 'We have heard really good things from patients about their treatment experiences and aftercare.' However, many participants did question the impact the local ISTC had had on the integration of care across the health system, especially because the centre treats certain cases and has no facility to deal with significant complications. 'I can't help but feel the exclusion criterion makes it a little bit clunky', said the same executive. Others felt that pressure to 'make money' led providers (NHS and non-NHS) to manipulate contracts in a way that was detrimental to quality:

> Providers seem only to use clinical evidence in service contracts when it is financially beneficial for them to do so. Provider priorities are not in easing care pathways or necessarily looking after patients' best interests.

4.5 Organisational efficiency up but questionable effects across the system

Organisational efficiency

In the respect that secondary care providers know they have to earn their income in order to continue operating, the market has made organisations more cost-conscious. In turn, this has helped to drive efficiency. As one medically-qualified executive put it:

> [The trust being a business] makes us think in a lean fashion. For example, we recently streamlined prosthesis and implants. It wasn't our preference, but doing it saved money without adversely affecting patient care. We have to be making money in our own patch. If we're not, we have to ask ourselves why, because other hospitals can make money on the tariff... You can't lose money this way in the real world, and you shouldn't be able to do it in the health service.

Another commented specifically on the increase in efficiency seen with the creation of FTs: 'I think the process... has been hugely beneficial. We were forced to really look in detail at internal processes and current strategies.'

At the organisational level, executives are increasingly seeing their role as similar to that of running a business or, as one participant (at a non-FT) put it, 'aiming to maximise revenue and efficiencies'. This is most clearly seen in reported decisions on service development and closures, where a lack of profitability was the most commonly given rationale. One provider executive said:

> We would stop an existing service if it were not profitable or if we did not have enough resources to run a decent service. The days of [all] hospitals doing everything is gone. We know we can't be good at everything because most disciplines are becoming increasingly specialised, and we only have so much capacity. Sometimes you have to give as well as take, build on your strengths and let go of your weaknesses, letting other hospitals do what they do best.

34

Another reported:

> As for deciding to provide something new, we first ask 'Is there a market opportunity for this service?' and then, 'Will we be able to meet the targets around the service?' and finally, 'Will it produce a surplus?'

Another, in describing his responsibility for stopping the 'creeping development' of services, which, despite being advocated by clinicians or PCTs, do not fit with the trust's wider business strategy, explained: 'If a service is financially non-viable, it's a no-go from the start.'

System-wide efficiency

Whether or not such 'business attitudes' have translated to benefits across the system, however, is unclear. Waiting times, for example, fell dramatically post-2002, but disagreement existed among interviewees on the extent to which the market was responsible. One medically-qualified executive reasoned:

> I've been a consultant for 13 years. Back when I started people waited 18 months for an operation and had no idea what was going on. Now the same [physician] sees them throughout, and they are turned around in 18 weeks. It's fantastic for patients as an end-user. [The market] is not a bad package.

Another commented:

> Waiting times have certainly improved in the region since [the ISTC] has been operating. It used to take two years to get an MRI [scan]!

Efficiency at new providers in our sample health economy was typically impressive. One interviewee, for example, documented how the diagnostics and treatment scheme makes the NHS a 24 per cent saving compared to the average cost of the same procedures if carried out in NHS providers, with patients seen quicker and making on average 1.6 fewer visits before diagnosis (1.2 *vis-à-vis* 2.8). Another PCT executive gave a further example of efficiency at newer, independent clinics, saying:

> ECG services were recently given to a private provider. Previously it was carried out in the hospital, [with] higher costs.

However, most participants felt that targets, rather than the market, had been more of a catalyst in causing waiting times to fall, with many pointing out that both the ISTC and diagnostics scheme are significantly under-utilised. 'We got a £30m white elephant', said one NHS provider executive.

Others focused on the impact of the market on the sustainability of the system as a whole, frequently referring to the incentives hospitals have to increase income and noting that although organisational efficiency may be increasing, sometimes hospitals are doing the wrong things more efficiently. One provider executive used data from the region in general, and his acute trust in particular, to illustrate this sentiment:

> About two or three years ago an audit was carried out of hospitals in the region, looking at re-admission following fracture in elderly people. In most hospitals, there was around a 35 per cent re-admission rate. At ours it was 80 per cent, because there are just no other facilities outside the hospital to support them.

There is little incentive under PbR for hospitals to reduce re-admissions because this would cause their revenue to fall. The same executive continued:

> At the moment, across a year, six per cent of our patients account for 49 per cent of bed days, with many frequent flyers readmitted six, seven, eight times a year. Predominantly they have COPD, angina, MI, UTI, falls and diabetes. We don't do care in the community properly. [There is no] automatic incentive to effectively manage a person's health care.

A PCT executive went so far as to say 'the current structure is bankrupting the system'.

4.6 Discussion

To return to our research question, what emerges from the findings presented in this chapter is that, by and large, the market in the NHS is yet to 1) have the full intended impact on the behaviour of secondary care provider organisations and 2) produce the expected benefits—improved quality, efficiency, innovation, responsiveness to customers, and equity—on any meaningful or systematic scale. There are isolated and subtle examples of the market having such effects. Providers in both our sample health economy and validation sites, for example, reported being more customer-focused; image-conscious; aware of the actions of others; made to 'think' when tenders are put out; and have, in more than a few cases, used the threat of losing business—even if more hypothetical than real—to motivate change internally. Organisations have also been forced to look harder at their operational efficiency.

However, such effects are far from the widespread benefits and changes in behaviour anticipated, or hoped for, by protagonists of the market. In most of the cases cited in the previous paragraph, there is a real debate to be had as to whether it is actually the *market*—in terms of the possibility of losing business through patients' choices over where to go for treatment, or PCT decisions to re-commission services—that has motivated change, or simply a desire to have a better public image than other local acute trusts (i.e. an effort to improve on published performance data). More widely, it is clear that there are many other factors that drive behaviour and performance in secondary care organisations. Although it is not possible to measure qualitatively the relative strength of any one causal factor to any degree of certainty, most executives we spoke to felt factors such as targets, a desire to achieve good CQC ratings, a culture of continuous quality improvement, and professional pride had far greater influence in driving performance than the threat of competition posed by the market. This is consistent with the findings of the majority academic studies on the market in the NHS to date, including the most recent by The King's Fund on patient choice.[1]

Perhaps this should come as no surprise. At the most fundamental level, to no significant extent has there been the basic changes in organisational behaviour that one would typically expect and rely on in a market environment (or at least a competitive one) to sharpen incentives: increased responsiveness to customers—in particular to PCTs as the local commissioners of care—and real concern about the activities and plans of others. With such changes absent, it is unrealistic to expect most of the benefits anticipated and routinely seen from markets in other industries—improved quality, efficiency, innovation, responsiveness to customers, and equity—to materialise. The canonical question, then, must be *why* haven't such changes in behaviour (and, in turn, performance) generally occurred? It is this question that we attempt to answer with the remainder of the book.

PART 2:

Why isn't the market delivering greater benefits?

5

Is the concept of a market in the NHS flawed?

To reiterate our core findings: by and large, the market in the NHS is yet to 1) have its intended impacts on the behaviour of secondary care providers and 2) bring about the benefits subsequently expected—improved quality, efficiency, innovation, responsiveness to customers, and equity—on any meaningful or systematic scale.

The key question is *why*? Here, the semi-structured approach we adopted throughout the interviews proved its value, giving participants the opportunity to expand extensively along the lines of questioning.[i] When interview scripts were analysed, coded and compared, this not only provided us with a powerful understanding as to *whether* the market is working, but also *how* the market is working (or not) and, consequently, *why* it is (or not). The previous chapter presented our findings on the first question of this triad. In the coming chapters we present our findings on the latter two—findings that we believe are crucial to guiding future policy direction relating to the market in the NHS.

In essence, the issues described by the participants—executives and clinicians at PCTs, NHS trusts, foundation trusts and practice-based commissioning groups—point to two possible scenarios:

1. The concept of a market operating in the NHS is flawed and therefore any attempt to introduce one is unlikely to be effective;

2. A market can be effective in the NHS, but it is not currently working because it is being distorted and/or stifled.

Clearly policy implications are drastically different depending on which scenario the balance of evidence supports. The latter suggests a need for 'tweaking' (though perhaps significantly in some places) and working more with what exists; the former suggests that fundamental

---

i   If it became clear to us in the course of the interviews that the participant thought market policies were not working as intended, we began to extend core questions to focus on why he or she felt this might be.

change, of one form or another, is a necessity if the NHS is to withstand the coming financial challenges.

The presentation and discussion of our findings with regard to the second scenario, that the market is being distorted and/or stifled, is reserved for the following chapter. In this chapter we focus on the first scenario: that the concept of a market operating in the NHS is flawed. Our findings are grouped under three headings:

1. PCTs consider levers other than those available through the market (i.e. competitive pressure resulting from the threat of losing business) to be more effective in driving the performance of secondary care providers;

2. Many theoretical problems with the application of markets in health care have manifested themselves in the NHS as a result of the introduction of a market;

3. The political and centralised nature of the NHS may forever quash market incentives.

In the discussion at the end of the chapter we analyse whether, combined, these findings represent such fundamental problems that the market should be abandoned, or whether they might be overcome.

5.1 The market is considered less effective than other means of driving performance in providers

a. Targets, quality initiatives and the open publication of information
As indicated in the discussion of the previous chapter's findings (see section 4.6), there are a number of other factors (internal and external) that influence the behaviour and performance of secondary care providers aside from market pressure. Many participants, at both providers and PCTs, felt these factors had more impact on decision-making in providers and were ultimately more effective ways to drive performance. This applied particularly to the effect of targets, pay-for-performance initiatives, and the open publication of information on performance. One PCT executive reported:

Our strongest lever is probably CQUIN,[ii] where we can reward acute trusts for their adherence to particular pathways, and the fact that we can refuse to pay if the acute trusts do not produce a discharge summary.

Another reasoned:

This attempt at making district general hospitals into entrepreneurial organisations has been a failure. It has not been successful in moving resources from secondary care to primary care. Within a publicly funded system, I think we can obtain the desired benefits of competition more reliably through good assessment techniques and benchmarking outcomes.

Some provider executives expressed sympathy with this view. 'Targets have been much more of a catalyst for us than local contestability', said one executive. Another, in one of our validation sites, stated:

For us, the prospect of losing a bit of activity at the margin is much less of a daily worry than losing two per cent of income based on meeting some quality metrics or targets. For example, a failure to do x for y patients under CQUIN could mean losing £0.5m, which is very noticeable.

Others focused on the power of intrinsic motivation. 'A lot of what is deemed competition can be attributed to chief executives' ambitions for their individual trusts', said one provider participant.

b. 'Preferred' providers, PCT self-provision and integrated care organisations
Also relevant is the fact that one or two PCTs in our sample health economy had apparently turned their backs on using the market. One executive reported:

Our PCT is a relatively old PCT. It has been in place longer than many others and has had the time to figure out what works and how to achieve stability. And the answer has not been competition [in terms of the threat of moving business elsewhere].

We found three practical (or structural) manifestations of this rejection of market structures. The first is a preference for working with a single ('preferred') provider rather than wielding the threat of taking business elsewhere. As one PCT executive put it:

---

ii   As referred to in previous chapters, Commissioning for Quality and Innovation (CQUIN) is a relatively new payment scheme that makes a proportion of providers' income conditional on agreed markers of quality and innovation.

I think the advantages are in the long term relationship, which allows us to, in a way, 'manage' the supplier. When our intent to purchase is clear, we have a continuity of engagement with the trust, and it enables an ongoing dialogue with heavy clinician input.

Other reasons given for working with a single provider were: the development of clinical pathways is more difficult in a market-based system; clinical governance processes are more easily agreed upon in a long-term, preferred provider-type partnership; and it is easier to undertake case investigations or carry out root-cause analyses where necessary because lines of communication are familiar.

Second, some (but by no means all) PCT executives expressed a preference for managing and providing services 'in-house' rather than going through tendering processes. One PCT executive reasoned:

It gives you the ability to change provision processes according to need, without having to spend time and resources on market testing.

Another stated:

You know, a year ago I would have said that PCTs need to completely devolve their provider arms, that it was a conflict of interest,[iii] but this year, after having started our own provision, I really think it is the way to go... everything is just much more connected, holistic and transparent when it is all in one space.[iv]

Third, a few PCTs are looking to take such collaborative relationships with providers further through creating 'integrated care organisations' that link certain elements of primary, secondary and community care services in pathways that offer, in the words of one provider executive, 'greater incentives [for hospitals] to collaborate instead of compete'. One participant described her PCT's intention, for example, to base such integration on the United States health maintenance organisation Kaiser Permanente's principles of prevention, early diagnosis and early discharge, arguing this could

---

iii   Because PCTs have the incentive to contract their provider arm before external providers, in order to keep funds 'in house'.

iv   Not all interviewees agreed with this. One PCT executive reported: 'Divesting PCTs of provider arms is the right thing to do. It narrows the breadth of our role and allows those who want to commission, to commission; and those that want to lead provision, to lead provision.'

44

improve quality and efficiency at a faster rate than the current market structure.[v]

5.2 Wider problems stemming from markets in health care

The preference for using structures and performance levers other than the market—such as integrated care organisations and targets—was not always based on a belief that they are more effective in changing provider behaviour. For some, the choice was driven by a view that the market is actually inhibiting improvement and is detrimental to quality of care. In this line of argument, participants drew particular attention to a number of market failures associated with health care that were alluded to in section 2.1.

a. Collaboration undermined

The majority of participants, from both PCTs and acute trusts, highlighted the importance of collaboration in medical care at some point in the interview, with a few referring to academic studies to support their case.[1] One provider executive commented:

> Medicine is not like producing Land Rovers. There are undoubtedly aspects [of medicine] which only work in a collaborative mechanism... and the greater complexity of medicine now demands greater complexity of partnership.

Many considered the (re-)introduction of the market in the NHS to have inhibited such partnership; they were more likely to describe relationships between purchasers and providers, and between providers themselves, as adversarial rather than collaborative. Executives were quick to blame others for problems, rather than to take joint responsibility. One provider executive stated:

> In an ideal world we would collaborate and talk to [a nearby hospital] about service pathways and such, but we don't communicate effectively as we are both positioning to become a single future centre, if there is one.

---

v   It should, however, be said that although Kaiser Permanente is an integrated care organisation, its executives typically attribute some of its success to the competitive pressure of operating in a market. Enthoven, A.C., 'Commentary: Competition made them do it', *BMJ* 2002; 324:135-143 (http://www.bmj.com/cgi/content/full/324/7330/135#resp3, accessed 27 July 2010).

Another reflected:

> Something happened with the introduction and roll out of the market reforms, which somehow discouraged this [clinician to clinician] type of communication.

In giving examples of worsening collaboration, attention was drawn to two particular interfaces of care. The first is the relationship between primary and secondary care. One provider executive commented:

> There are organisational and clinical governance problems resulting from the purchaser/provider split [the basis of the market], and it hasn't been done in the interests of patients. There are no real relationships between primary and secondary care. There is no reliable quality assurance.

A PCT executive described an example of this:

> FTs can choose to [cooperate] when it suits them. Take MRSA de-colonisation as an example; it's not in anyone's contract as to what to do. So FTs will often refer patients back to their GP; and then the GP will say it's not their responsibility.

The second example relates to the introduction of new providers, which some felt interrupts long term investment in clinical pathways within the NHS and creates obstacles to communication. 'There are a lot of safety issues to consider. Patients are constantly seeing different doctors', said one medically-qualified provider executive. A PCT executive argued:

> We need policies that will pull us together and encourage collaboration. In some senses market policies make you feel as though you are not in it together, and that's not what we need to get through the years ahead.

b. Wasted resources

Participants raised two associated concerns over waste emerging in the NHS as a result of the market environment. The overriding concern was that the market encourages unnecessary duplication and the keeping of excess capacity that the NHS cannot afford.[vi] One PCT executive put it as such:

> The NHS is structured not to have any excess capacity or inefficiencies. But a real market requires providers to operate at far less than 100 per cent capacity so that purchasers can actually choose to switch between them. However, how can

---

vi   This point may be questioned. Markets do need excess capacity but the question is whether the existence of it—and the competition it facilitates—spurs providers to be more efficient than if it was not there.

we justify providing any excess capacity when the system is run with public funds?

The most frequent example given of this (aside from the afore-mentioned issues surrounding ISTCs, see section 4.5), is the incentive the market provides for hospitals within the same region to develop the very same, expensive, speciality services. The provider above, who mentioned the lack of communication between his and another large, nearby hospital, also made this point:

> There is some conflict over which specialty services each of us will provide. For example, [one FT] runs a cardiac surgery centre, as does [ours]. I would say we each have an equal market share in cardiac surgery. But [our region] doesn't need two big heart centres in such close proximity...

Others questioned the very logic of having a market when it comes to such services. One PCT executive argued:

> Some services are so niche or so expensive to start up that it's hard for new providers to enter the market, for example, neurosurgery.

The second concern was that the market, in encouraging providers to continuously increase activity in order to maximise income, creates unnecessary tension in a system that by its nature is operating with a finite budget. One PCT executive opined:

> A market is a very specific thing where producers want to continuously increase consumer transactions—but we actually don't want people overusing GP and acute care.

Another PCT executive described the perceived consequences in more vitriolic terms: 'FTs can turn a surplus when the rest of the [health] economy is in meltdown.'

c. Uninformed and ineffective consumers

Turning now to the 'demand' side of the market, one implication is that (at least for electives where patients have a choice of provider at the point of referral) patients are no longer just 'patients', but are also encouraged to be 'consumers' or 'customers'. Participants felt this created two prob-lems. The first relates to a specific market failure identified in section 2.1, that of asymmetric information between providers and 'consumers'. Most interviewees felt patients either did not have enough information to choose effectively (particularly on the basis of quality), or could not understand the information available. One PCT executive commented: 'Patients' criteria for choice are often not based on knowledge of outcomes [of care] but on convenience.'

A provider executive explained:

> We try to get the message out that we have lower MRSA, C-diff and waiting times than other trusts... but the public's impression is probably still that [they] are better. New, gleaming buildings somehow builds confidence. Most of the public take clinical excellence in quality as standard, even if they shouldn't, and instead differentiate hospitals by such things as car parking, buildings and the food.

A few participants additionally felt patient choice fragmented pathways of care. They argued that PCTs would be better able to ensure high quality care if allowed to direct patients to the providers they (PCTs) deemed to be the best, and concentrate on building strong pathways of care (including discharge arrangements etc) around these.

The second concern was that introducing a market within a publicly-funded system that is free-at-the-point-of-use is encouraging irresponsible behaviour by patients. As one PCT executive reported:

> Patients are encouraged to be consumers without having to actually spend any money, which has negative effects on individual responsibility.

A provider executive provided an example of this:

> The threshold for demand has been lowered. Patients, who, prior to the enforcement of the national four-hour A&E waiting target, may have decided a problem was too minor to warrant a visit, may now rationalise: 'Why not go to the A&E? I am guaranteed to be seen in four hours'.

d. Profits before patients

Drawing together the findings of this sub-section, some participants felt that the overriding need for providers to find ways to survive in the market and satisfy customers was having detrimental effects on quality of care. This concern was expressed particularly in reference to the impact of the market on 1) the ability of PCTs to ensure the right services are available and 2) day-to-day decision-making in providers. On the former, one PCT executive said:

> With [the market] the way it is, there are problems in understanding who is doing what and what they are not doing. If an FT finds a service is not making

money, they may decide to close it down. If all [nearby FTs] make similar decisions, there is going to be a major gap in local treatment.

Along similar lines, one provider executive, when asked what is considered first when deciding to develop a new service at the trust, replied: 'I see what you are getting at, and the honest answer is, it's not always the patient.'

Looking at the latter point, concerning day-to-day decision-making in providers, executives at both PCTs and providers described examples of acute trusts 'gaming' the system to increase activity and—through the payment-by-results framework—income. Such decisions included: unnecessarily admitting patients who present through A&E; conducting consultant-to-consultant referrals 'out of proportion with patient need'; and keeping patients in hospital longer than necessary. One PCT executive opined:

Figuratively, [PbR] gives providers a way of printing money. They can earn more for poor clinical decisions.

Another said:

It isn't payment by results; it's payment by activity, so from the hospitals' point of view, the more activity the better.

Provider executives, too, expressed some sympathy with this view. 'I can see where PCTs are coming from', one said '[Payment-by-results does create] a bit of an endless quest for spurious accuracy.'

5.3 Political and centralised nature of the NHS may forever quash market incentives

Setting aside concerns around market failure, a further problem presented by a few participants was that the political and centralised nature of the NHS may in fact forever work against a market being effective. One interviewee observed:

Markets do not align themselves with political timescales, and this poses the problem that governments looking for politically helpful outcomes find that markets usually fail to deliver the goods to fit in nicely with elections and manifestos.

A few felt this was at least part of the reason why other means to drive performance, such as targets and pay-for-performance initiatives, had been more effective than market pressures. As one provider executive reflected, 'You can't really be left to manage your own business as a trust without first satisfying what the DH requires.'

Another said:

[In a market] providers need to recognise the future benefit of a current investment, even though it might not produce short-term gain. [But] it is difficult to convince the NHS to change its ways, especially as providers are assessed and rewarded on an annual (or three-year) basis.

Delving into the detail, we found three manifestations of conflicts between the political and centralised nature of the NHS and having a market: constantly changing policy; government targets; and unwillingness to allow for hospital closures. Here, we examine each in turn.

a. Constantly changing policy

Throughout the interviews executives at providers and (especially) PCTs frequently expressed bewilderment over the constantly changing focus of government policy, particularly with regard to the market. One provider executive explained:

We all need to know when we are to be competing and when we are to be collaborating. There is often a very blurred line, and it's not communicated enough either from the DH or between providers.

At the time we carried out the interviews for this study, for example, the then Labour Government had recently announced that, in contradiction to the same Government's *Principles and Rules for Cooperation and Competition*[2(vii)] for the NHS, PCTs were to consider NHS organisations as their 'preferred providers' of services.[3] While some executives were inclined to ignore the change (dismissing it as 'political speak'), others expressed puzzlement ('does anyone really know what

---

vii In an annex to the NHS Operating Framework for 2008/09, the government had sort to clarify the situation around the market in the NHS by publishing a relatively short (16 page) document that set out the guiding principles for the market; the rationale behind the principles; expected actions and behaviours; and rules to be followed. The number one principle was that 'Commissioners should commission services from the providers who are best placed to deliver the needs of their patients and population'. These later formed the terms of reference for the Cooperation and Competition Panel (CCP), formed in 2009 to 'investigate and advise the DH and Monitor on potential breaches', relating to conduct, mergers, procurement and advertising.

that means?') and others acted on it directly (for example, by pro-hibiting independent providers from responding to tenders). One PCT executive commented:

> We were never the sort of PCT where tendering was preferred anyway and we were just at the point of beginning to put services out to tender, when now the default is the opposite. It seems the market is dead.

More broadly, participants referred to at least four (negative) consequences of such constant change. First, that attention of organisations is diverted to conforming with the latest policy or structural reorganisation and away from improving processes of care. Second, that it is difficult for PCTs and providers to make meaningful comparisons of performance year-on-year, because structures and processes have often changed. Third, that due to the risk of policy changes, particularly those that may move the NHS away from a market, independent and voluntary sector providers are reluctant to invest for the medium and long-term. Fourth, that constant change often results in a web of conflicting goals and incentives for organisations, as bits and pieces of different policies are left in place without full consideration of the impact on new ones. Summing up the situation, one provider executive reflected 'all of the energy put toward working out what we are supposed to be doing regarding [the market] could actually be put to much better use'.

b. Government targets

As emphasised in section 2.1, for a market to be effective, participants generally require a certain freedom of action in order to respond to the needs of consumers and to have the time and resources to devote to innovating and improving services. In the view of some participants, however, such freedom of action is severely curtailed in the NHS by the continued attention of the government to directing the state of play, and setting and monitoring targets. Three consequences of the latter were noted. First, many participants felt the bureaucracy associated with targets is time-consuming and encourages short-term attitudes, which are not conducive to innovation. One PCT executive reported:

> There are also just too many targets; we are being checked to death... Naturally programmes with long-term benefits will take a back seat.

51

Another said:

> There is an absurd amount of regulation in health care. We barely have time to concentrate on our jobs because there are so many processes to follow and organisations to report to.

Second, a few commented that the environment that targets and central direction tend to create is not conducive to organisations taking the initiative (as is required in a market). One provider executive opined: 'The DH has a tendency to tell everyone how exactly to do things, instead of telling organisations what its goals are and letting us figure out the best ways to reach them.' A PbC executive expressed similar sentiment: 'the amount of guidance... leaves us little discretion in the way we do things'.

Third, participants felt targets can distract attention toward activities that may not be productive. One provider executive reported: '...right now the contracts and negotiations [with PCTs] are mostly focused on ticking boxes and meeting targets [rather than focusing on the patient]'. Another drew attention to the impact of the World Class Commissioning (WCC) assurance regime (the DH-led system intended to ensure PCTs can competently commission) in 'directing' the market:

> [We] need a massive effort to sort out pathways so that [we] buy the right thing. [But] WCC doesn't do this; in fact you can buy rubbish as a commissioner and be 'world class' under WCC!

c. Unwillingness to accept hospital closures
This is a brief but important point that exemplifies the dichotomy posed by the government's continued ownership of and responsibility for the NHS, and the introduction of a market. As outlined in section 2.1, a defining feature of markets is that organisations can fail. However, a few interviewees referred to a significant contradiction between this and the reluctance of any government to countenance hospitals closing or being taken over, often for fear of harming the NHS 'brand'. In the words of one PCT executive: 'We can't afford, politically, to shut down a hospital, however bad it is.' Another reported (for the same reason): 'We can't put competition against a failing district general hospital (DGH).'

5.4 Discussion

In this section we have presented findings in support of the argument that the market in the NHS has yet to have its intended impact on secondary care providers and produce the expected benefits because the concept of a market operating in the NHS is, in fact, flawed and thus unlikely to ever be effective.

There is evidence to support this argument. To reiterate, participants referred to numerous occasions when they considered other means, such as the pressure of targets and pay-for-performance programmes, had been more effective in driving provider performance than the market (i.e. the threat of losing business). A few also suggested the market could, in fact, be detrimental to high quality care in describing the consequences of a number of market failures and they presented evidence that, regardless of this, the political and centralised nature of the NHS may forever work against a market being effective. Perhaps the most powerful point is the first one. If other factors are considered more effective than market pressure in changing behaviours and motivating secondary care providers, we may question why we should risk all the costs associated with market failure and spend time trying to settle the conflict between the political nature of the NHS and the autonomy needed for a market to function. Indeed, previous research does show that—consistent with our findings—targets have probably been more of a catalyst for improved performance in the NHS over the past decade than the market,[4] and that encouraging competition through the open publication of performance data, rather than a market for service provision, can be a significant driver of quality.[5]

However, we do not feel our findings are robust enough to support the underlying thesis of this chapter.

a. What market?

Some of the most abundant evidence emerging from our research related not to the effectiveness of the market within the NHS, but instead to whether or not there is actually a market to analyse, in the respect of there being meaningful competitive pressure on organisations. Evidence summarised by the Office of Fair Trading shows that one cannot expect a market to deliver significant benefits unless there is, in fact, sufficient threat of losing business (i.e. sufficient that providers operate on the assumption that losing—and gaining—business is a real possibility).[6(viii)] Yet, as we saw in Chapter 4, few providers considered the actions of others in developing strategy or considered it particularly important to be responsive to commissioners (PCTs, patients or PbC groups). According to participants, patients in their area have thus far proved reluctant consumers (or have not been given enough information), and PCTs reluctant commissioners.[(ix)] It is thus reasonable to ask whether interviewees can be certain that market mechanisms are less effective than other means of driving secondary care performance, for the simple reason that the market that was intended for the NHS has not been truly implemented. In addition to this—as we shall see in Chapter 6—many concerns highlighted by participants and linked by them to the market can be attributed to the market's immaturity. For example, markets can, and do, facilitate collaborative relationships, particularly between buyers and sellers, as well as competition. And where competition is real, the existence of excess capacity can fuel greater efficiency than if there was none.

b. Market mechanisms, even in their current form, have still had impact
Additionally, and conceding the above point that previous research supports our finding that other levers have thus far had a greater effect than market mechanisms in driving performance in secondary care, the most recent studies on the market in the NHS do show the market having certain positive effects. As documented in section 2.5, they indicate the market has: improved managerial quality; reduced

---

[viii] This does not necessarily require a lot of 'switching', but that providers *believe* the threat of switching is real. Consider network providers in the mobile phone industry. Competition is rife, and innovations are quickly copied out of fear of losing business (which is a very real possibility and would almost certainly happen if innovations were not copied).

[ix] In our sample health economy just over half of elective care referrals were made through Choose and Book (which facilitates patient choice) as of November 2009, with around 3.5 per cent of *all* referrals going to private providers; and, while all three PCTs interviewed had increased the number of community and non-acute service contracts for which providers could compete (with one PCT putting six services out to tender in the past year), all were small in scope and budget, so even when taken away from existing NHS providers the contracts had little impact on overall income.

inequalities in access (in terms of waiting times); improved quality as measured by 30-day in-hospital mortality from acute myocardial infarction; and reduced length-of-stay.[7] Nor should we forget the core findings of this study, for although we did not find the market in the NHS to be by and large 1) impacting the behaviour of secondary care providers as intended and 2) driving the expected benefits in patient care on any meaningful or systematic scale, we did find instances in which, despite the absence of a truly functioning market, these outcomes were evident and attributed to market pressures by participants.[x]

c. Support for the market structure

For most of the individual arguments put against the use of market mechanisms reported in this chapter, there are counter-arguments which were often dually expressed by participants in interviews. On the first point presented — that other levers are more effective in driving performance than the market — even those who criticised the market quite stridently tended to support the foundations of it: the split between purchasers and providers. Typically, this was on the basis that it is useful to have a means (PCTs) through which a) population and patient interests can be represented independently of professional or organisational interests and b) resources can be effectively matched with need. Additionally, most PCT executives acknowledged the value of having the ability to take business elsewhere, even if it is a last resort and even if (as is likely) it is not appropriate in all circumstances.[xi] As one said:

> For me the market in the NHS currently is the concept that providers of NHS services cannot assume the right to provide irrespective of the views of patients... i.e. whether or not there is 'real' competition in terms of consumer switching or active decommissioning of services, providers cannot assume (with

---

[x] Nor should we forget the imperfections in other means to drive performance, such as central direction; professionalism; and democratic means (or increased 'voice' for patients).

[xi] Others were more strident. One said: 'The only lever we really have is the threat of competition, [that] providers know that we could actually purchase elsewhere.'

the exception of very few highly specialist services) that they will be the provider of care forever.

To summarise, while there is some evidence to suggest that the market is not yet delivering benefits because a market can never be effective in the NHS, the evidence is by no means conclusive. This is not least because the majority of findings discussed in this chapter can also be explained by the fact that the market for secondary care which was intended for the NHS has not been truly implemented. We turn now to this alternative thesis: that the NHS has not seen the anticipated impacts on the behaviour and performance of secondary care providers because the implementation of the market is being distorted or stifled.

6

Is the market being distorted and stifled?

In the previous chapter we began to consider possible explanations for our core findings (that the market is yet to 1) have the intended impact on the behaviour of secondary care providers and 2) drive the expected benefits—improved quality, efficiency, innovation, responsiveness to customers, and equity—on any meaningful or systematic scale) by looking at whether the market is conceptually flawed and, thus, unlikely to ever be effective. Doubt was cast on this thesis not least because: first, we did not see enough evidence that the market has been sufficiently implemented for such a conclusion to be drawn (a fact that, in itself, could explain some of the negative consequences of the market detailed by participants[i]); and second, although we found examples of negative effects, participants did report some examples of the benefits anticipated. The latter point alone raises the question: if markets are by nature incompatible with the NHS, why would we see any associated increases in innovation or efficiency at all?

In this chapter we review our findings in support of an alternative explanation: that the market in the NHS is failing to drive performance to the extent anticipated less because it cannot do so, more because it is being distorted and/or stifled. Indeed, the most commonly recurring theme in our analysis was the existence of numerous barriers— structural, practical, political and cultural—that are preventing market policies from operating as intended.

In Part A below, we focus on apparent distortions in the current structure of the market, while in Part B we focus on other, non-structural, factors and influences that seem to be stifling or preventing the market from working. After each part we discuss the implications of our findings.

---

i   For example, there is a case to be made that acute trusts have been able to dictate terms to PCTs and patients (their 'customers'), precisely because they do not see the threat of losing business as real.

PART A: Distortions in the market

In the course of the previous chapter—in discussing the impact of the political and centralised nature of the NHS—we referred to the impact of government targets. This, in fact, also provides the first example of a distorting influence on the market which, some participants felt, forces it to work in unintended ways, encouraging providers to 'compete' over meeting targets, rather than on many other standards shown to be valued by patients and purchasers through fluctuations of supply and demand (see section 5.3b). In the current section, we focus on additional structural concerns across the NHS that appear to be having the same effect: distorting the intended impact of the market on the behaviour of secondary care providers, and therefore restricting anticipated benefits. These are as follows: an imbalance of power between purchasers and providers; an uneven playing field between NHS and non-NHS providers; problems with payment-by-results; and the role of GPs.

6A.1. Structural imbalance of power between purchasers and providers

As documented in our core findings (section 4.1), we did not find much evidence of an increase in responsiveness of providers to purchasers—patients, PCTs and practice-based commissioners—that one would expect in a market. In fact, as the main purchasers of care, PCTs seemed to have limited ability to exert influence over providers, to promote patient choice, and to switch services (where necessary) to secure improvements in health care. Participants referred to three structural concerns that help explain PCTs' weak position: PCTs are too small *vis-à-vis* providers; acute trusts are more established organisations within the healthcare system; and PbC—typically PCTs' strongest link to clinicians—is often not well supported.

a. PCTs are too small relative to providers

The argument that PCTs are 'too small' was typically expressed by participants in relation to two things. The first is that PCTs do not have enough resources to devote to developing markets and building the requisite skills to commission effectively across the spectrum of care—particularly given the broad range of responsibilities they have. One PCT executive explained: 'The agenda set out for providers seems manageable, but ours stretches resources too thin and prevents us from investing in areas we really need to—namely procurement and contracting.' An SHA executive commented on one consequence of this, in relation to the lack of influence of PCTs over providers:

> I've no doubt if you're asking PCTs to be expert commissioners in every subject area they will come out looking stupid, because they can't do it... a £40k p.a. PCT worker in front of a cardiology manager will be made into mincemeat.

The second point often put forward was that individual PCTs, because of their size, simply have too little bargaining power *vis-à-vis* acute trusts. As one PCT executive put it:

> We are the xth largest PCT in the country, and we still don't have enough bargaining power. I can't imagine what it must be like for smaller PCTs.

A PbC executive similarly reflected: '[PCTs] do not have enough pull in the relationship to effectively do their jobs—to commission for patient benefit.'

Provider executives tended to concur on the disadvantages of PCTs' size and expressed irritation at the subsequently large number of purchasing organisations their trusts must negotiate with. One argued:

> Regional commissioning could be consolidated and streamlined, which would make it easier for providers to plan. It is currently quite patchy and inconsistent.

For precisely such reasons, there are currently efforts to develop associations that aim to pool knowledge, commission low volume services on behalf of multiple PCTs, and help develop procurement skills in both our sample health economy and one of our study's validation areas. One official from a validation site described the reasoning as follows:

> PCTs recognise the need and benefit in aggregating commissioning to counter-balance the power of heavyweight [provider] organisations. A combined budget [of one billion pounds plus] is significantly greater than an individual one.

b. Acute trusts are more established in the health system

Compared with the majority of acute trusts, PCTs are relatively new entities. Participants felt this afforded acute trusts a number of advantages, namely that they: have clinicians 'right there, involved in decisions, pushing for what they want'; have the 'patients onside' because 'people don't know what PCTs are'; and have closer, historical links with the DH.

A large number of interviewees felt the DH and government were, as a result, more receptive to acute trusts' concerns than those of PCTs. One PCT executive gave the example of a continued tendency on the part of the DH to consult acute trusts on policy changes before PCTs:

> This means the hospitals often know in advance what is coming and are able to plan for it... This happened with HRG4 [changes to the payment-by-results tariff]. When PCTs were finally shown the contract, we were given only two months to sign. The hospitals had seen it much earlier and were able to plan their budgets for the following year. They knew about our deadline, so they refused to negotiate and simply let the time pass. HRG4 confused us and we lost millions of pounds.

This was corroborated by one official at the DH, who, unprompted, said:

> Commissioners are underpowered because until recently commissioning has not been given a high profile. The DH made the mistake of going straight to providers if there was a performance issue, which undermined PCTs.

A few PCT executives felt this trend has been exacerbated by the presence of a high-profile national regulator on the provider side, in the foundation trust regulator Monitor, and the absence of one on the commissioning side. One executive said:

> I think that FT relationships with PCTs get woollied by the presence of Monitor. Who is it that they are accountable to? In their eyes, definitely Monitor.

c. Practice-based commissioners are underpowered

In our sample health economy, PbC groups—which functioned as semi-autonomous work groups of the PCT—felt existing structures within the NHS afford them little real influence, leaving a feeling of frustration and disempowerment. Three concerns were particularly evident.

First, the groups claimed to be unable to make major changes to services because most of the providers they worked with held three-year contracts with PCTs that could only be altered after 'prohibitively long' arbitration processes (contracts which they also felt had been made with little clinical rigour).

Second, most PbC executives felt—perhaps because of this—that they had little influence when dealing with large acute trusts. One gave an example:

> The evidence exists that re-entry into the hospital system [for follow-up appointments for prostate cancer] does not bring additional benefits for

patients. The PbC hub is attempting to get hospital urologists to agree to a certain set of criteria for re-referral, in order to decrease costly outpatient attendances that may have otherwise been followed up in primary or community care. So far the provider will not formally agree.

And third, a few argued it was difficult to recruit GPs to engage with PbC generally. One stated:

> The incentives to participate are not strong enough. The only lure right now is a strong enough desire to improve care. Why should GPs want to be businessmen... especially when they are not receiving direct financial benefit?

One group had tried to combat this by obtaining legal status, which, one PbC executive argued, both creates stronger incentives for participation and creates greater leverage with providers:

> [It] obliges GPs to work together for the whole population they serve and provides inter-practice leverage. [We have now] been able to enforce a change in discharge letter procedure from [the main acute provider] back to the GPs. We regularly meet with the medical director, and I think our legal status gives us clout.

However, there were more fundamental disagreements among participants over whether practice-based commissioning, and indeed any form of GP-led commissioning, is structurally sound when it comes to administering a market in the NHS (see section 6A.4).

6A.2. Uneven playing field

As documented in section 2.1, markets are typically at their most effective when providers have as few *artificial* advantages over one another as possible (artificial advantages, not advantages derived from being more productive or offering a better service). However, none of our interviewees believed there was a level playing field between NHS and private/voluntary sector providers in this respect. For services tendered directly by PCTs (i.e. all except those negotiated nationally by the DH for ISTCs), interviewees referred to a number of factors that distort the market in NHS providers' favour.[ii] These included:

---

ii   The Office of Health Economics estimates that, on balance, there is a c. 14 per cent artificial cost advantage for NHS providers.

- **Pensions** are required to be 'fully funded' in the private/voluntary sectors, whereas the NHS pension scheme is funded primarily through state contributions, making labour costs cheaper for NHS organisations. Access to the NHS pensions scheme also creates powerful incentives for staff not to leave NHS providers for private or voluntary sector ones;

- **Capital costs** are lower for NHS providers where they have access to lending from HM Treasury;

- **The tax burden** on private sector providers is higher; they must pay VAT on services contracted-out and on seconded staff, and, due to the fact that costs and revenues are not treated symmetrically in the NHS and private sector, private sector providers face additional corporation tax;

- **Barriers to exit for failing NHS organisations** are significant. NHS providers are often supported financially and kept in the market artificially due to public/political resistance, regardless of their quality and efficiency relative to other providers;

- **Collusion among incumbent NHS providers**, both between acute trusts, and between GPs and acute trusts. This can and does block access to the market for private and voluntary providers (see section 6B.1);

- **The bureaucratic nature of tendering processes** typically followed by PCTs and the DH deters market entry (see section 6B.1, for a more detailed discussion). Disproportionate bid costs for small value contracts; tenders seeking replication of what is already done rather than inviting innovation; and over-prescriptive contracts, tend to discourage smaller providers from bidding for contracts (particularly from the voluntary sector).

Looking at the overall impact of cost advantages enjoyed by NHS providers, one PCT executive commented:

> It's always amusing and ironic when some NHS acute care providers try to argue that there is [an advantage for the private sector], but they [NHS providers] truly have so many means to thwart things back in their favour.

By way of contrast, however, more than a few executives felt the market was distorted the other way, i.e. towards private and voluntary sector providers when discussing nationally-negotiated ISTC contracts. Under these contracts, to stimulate the market, private sector providers were paid above the payment-by-results tariff, with guaranteed payment and defined case-mixes. One PCT executive detailed:

> These were centrally negotiated contracts, they were made by the DH on behalf of PCTs... then we were left to manage them... PCTs felt a bit imposed on and left out of the planning. They were quite woolly, weak contracts that left a lot of discretion to the ISTCs regarding who they would and would not treat. They could discharge sick patients whenever they liked, and those patients then became the responsibility of the NHS.

6A.3. Problems with payment-by-results

One of the most common complaints interviewees had about the current structure of the market related to the payment-by-results (PbR) framework through which secondary care providers are remunerated. In section 5.2d we described PbR as a potential source of tension between purchasers and providers in that it tends to incentivise increased hospital activity.[iii] In addition to this, many participants felt it distorts the market and restricts the market's potential to drive improvement in care through two means: 1) requiring payment be made per episode of care, even in cases where this might be inappropriate, and 2) ruling out price flexibility (under PbR prices are fixed).

On the first point, participants tended to focus on the use of PbR in paying for non-elective care, especially that concerned with chronic conditions. One provider executive explained the potential for negative consequences:

> PbR [for non-electives] is a good policy for hospitals, but not so much for patients... If we prevent an admission by good quality care, we lose money.

PCT executives tended to have the same opinion. One said:

---

iii PbR is a tariff system, under which providers are paid a flat rate (adjusted for a market forces factor) per procedure carried out, as opposed to a block contract for the year. It was introduced primarily to give providers the incentive to increase the number of elective patients treated, with the aim of reducing waiting times and encouraging providers to be more efficient.

The current system is not conducive to looking at supply chain pathways [when it comes to the management of chronic conditions] and wastage, which we need to be doing... PbR for non-electives has had its day and we are looking at options to replace it as soon as possible. It makes cooperation [between the PCT and hospitals] quite hard.

This is because PbR currently gives hospitals stronger financial incentives to, for example, carry on admitting patients with chronic conditions when complications arise (because they get paid per case), without necessarily focusing on better long-term management of such conditions in the home and community—which should, in turn, reduce unnecessary hospital admissions.

Turning to the second point, a few executives also felt the price rigidity inherent in payment-by-results (through there being a uniform tariff for each given procedure) works against an effective market because it prevents more efficient and innovative providers from passing on the benefit to commissioners in the form of lower prices and different 'products' (services). Others, too, questioned the transparency and means by which the tariff is derived. One PCT executive explained:

Right now commissioners are paying the same prices for vastly different outcomes. If providers were able to market services by offering different prices, commissioners could make more informed decisions on value for money.

Five PCT executives felt price flexibility, in particular, would offer a way out of the aforementioned conundrum presented by the use of payment-by-results for non-elective care. In the words of one participant, it would replace a 'rigid contract' with 'better tools', such as the ability to develop integrated payment for chronic conditions.

6A.4. The role of GPs

Although the focus of our study was on the market for secondary care, the role of GPs as 'gatekeepers' to secondary care and as practice-based commissioners is both important and impossible to ignore. Significantly, many interviewees felt this role was both ill-defined and lacking accountability, leading to significant distortions in the way the market operates.

Let us first consider GPs as 'gatekeepers'. On this, interviewees highlighted two related problems: 1) GPs bear no financial consequence for referral decisions and 2) for the most part GPs operate under the national General Medical Services contract, which PCTs are unable to directly influence. One provider executive reflected on the implications of this arrangement:

> PCTs need to figure out a way to control GP referrals. GPs are essentially independent contractors, yet the PCTs are responsible for the allocation of the funding that follows the patients... Referral ratios right now can vary from 1 to 100 [in our region] by individual GPs.

A PCT executive described a sense of powerlessness in working with GPs, due to their lack of contractual responsibility:

> [GPs] are independent contractors and don't want to be told by the PCTs how to make their referral decisions. They have loyalties, often to where they were trained. GPs don't seem to realise that their referrals are trigger points for monetary flow through the system.

This presents difficulties for PCTs in making decisions to commission services from different providers. One participant explained:

> It takes a while to switch the market, because GPs must [also] switch. Here, there are a lot of behavioural factors at play; if your GP annoys the local hip surgeon, he may be less willing to return his call about a patient at 3pm on a Sunday afternoon.

We turn now to the other role of GPs in the NHS, as practice-based commissioners. Interviewees criticised this on two opposing fronts. For some, PbC does not confer enough responsibility for commissioning to GPs. One PCT executive, for example, contrasted PbC with the internal market of the 1990s in which GPs held hard budgets to purchase elective care as 'GP fundholders'. He felt this created a greater alignment between financial consequence and the decisions to refer, and brought the market closer to patients than under current PbC arrangements.[iv]

For other participants, however, PbC—and any specific role for GPs in commissioning—represents something of a flawed model. One provider executive opined:

> How can GPs act as both commissioners and providers? They receive financial incentives [to refer patients to services they provide themselves], which makes

---

iv   In that savings could be re-invested by GP fundholders in other aspects of care. In PbC budgets are only indicative, and predominantly concerned with community care.

the process a complete conflict of interest. It's bad economics and can also be harmful to patients.

Another provider executive interviewed as part of our validation process put it as such:

> The government screwed up [the market] by allowing GPs and PCTs [traditionally providers of primary and community care] to be commissioners. Immediately you have the wrong type of competition, because they have the money, the incentive to pay it to themselves and to fight acute trusts over market share... It's like setting up a football team and asking the forwards to fight the defence [on the same team].

In other words such participants felt GP commissioning creates distortions in the market by conflating GPs' 'self-interest' in running general practice (which are independent businesses contracted to the NHS), and a role as 'impartial' commissioners on behalf of patients.

6A.5. Discussion

The distortions presented in this section clearly show that there is an alternative explanation for our core findings, i.e. why the market in the NHS has thus far failed to 1) have the intended impact on the behaviour of secondary care providers and 2) drive the expected benefits—improved quality, efficiency, innovation, responsiveness to customers, and equity—on any meaningful or systematic scale. The argument of the previous chapter—that the possibility of a functioning market within the NHS is conceptually flawed must be qualified by the fact that there are also a number of distortions apparently inhibiting the market's effectiveness.

It is worth returning to the theory presented in our background section (section 2.1). Here, we explained how (nearly) all markets require careful attention to structure and regulation to work effectively and how this is particularly so within public services, where: there are often a number of market failures; wider policy goals exist; and consumers do not generally pay directly for the service they receive.[1] Considering the findings presented in this section, it may well be the case that the structures and incentives plumbed for in the NHS are not the right ones for the market to be successful. Using the framework outlined by the Office of Fair Trading for successful markets in public services (see 2.1)[2] there appears to be: structural imbalance inhibiting the ability of purchasers (patients, PCTs and practice-based commissioners) to effectively influence providers; significant obstacles to real diversity in supply (due to the lack of a level playing field between NHS and non-NHS providers); and unhelpful distortions in funding and incentives stemming from targets, payment-by-results and GP-led commissioning. Addressing these may well lead to a more effective market.

However, this should be qualified on the basis of the strength of certain points raised by interviewees. Taking each point in turn:

1. There is a structural imbalance between purchasers and providers, but PCTs still hold the 'purse strings' and do have the ability to switch services between providers. The fact that by and large they have not done so is not wholly explained by any structural imbalance, nor is the fact that patients, for the most part, have not used their ability to choose providers at the point of referral;

2. There is an uneven playing field between NHS and non-NHS providers for routine tenders put out by PCTs, but there are factors that run in favour of non-NHS providers, not least the fact that they do not bear responsibility for training. Overall, however, the Office of Health Economics estimates NHS providers have a 14 per cent artificial cost advantage that should be ironed out;[3]

3. Government targets have distorted the focus of market activity—in that they focus provider attention on pre-decided issues as opposed to letting demand dictate the aspects of service customers want improved—however, it is well recognised that markets in health care are likely to under-provide information to patients, and that governments may need to mandate publication of relevant information.[4] Targets are one way of doing this. The problem may lie more in the fact that targets have primarily focused on waiting times and not—until recently with the CQUIN scheme—clinical outcomes;

4. There is reasonable evidence questioning the effectiveness of the payment-by-results tariff for non-elective care—a fact recognised by the DH in the 2010/11 Operating Framework, which announces work on the development of more integrated payment mechanisms in this area.[5] However, allowing price flexibility may not be the

optimum course because the fixed tariff is based on academic evidence suggesting competition is more likely to improve outcomes when prices are not allowed to vary (probably due to the difficulty of measuring outcomes in health care, and assigning causality as to why they vary);[6]

5. There are conflicts of interest and problems with accountability in practice-based commissioning and any GP-led commissioning. However, in compiling the evidence on the success of GP fundholding in the 1990s internal market (where GPs held hard budgets, rather than virtual ones as things currently stand), The King's Fund think-tank concluded GP fundholding was 'the most promising' of the 1990s reforms in terms of improving the quality and responsiveness of secondary care providers (though it was acknowledged that the evidence linking the policy to these outcomes was weak, particularly because GP fundholders were self-selected and enthusiastic about the policy).[7] It is likely that GP-led commissioning is neither a catch-all solution nor a catch-all problem, so long as lines of accountability are clearly and properly administered.

In summary, while there are structural distortions that may help to explain why the market in secondary care is not delivering the changes in behaviour and benefits that were anticipated, the explanation is not sufficient on its own. While the imbalance of power between purchasers and providers and the lack of a level playing field, for example, certainly make a functioning market difficult, the current structure is not so distortionary as to prevent PCTs from putting services out to tender and prevent hospitals from making changes to attract patients and commissioned services, for example. With this in mind, we turn now to factors referred to by participants that seem to be stifling the market's intended impact.

PART B. Stifling influences in the market

To reiterate, we have, thus far, considered two possible reasons as to why the market in the NHS, by and large, is yet to have its intended impact on secondary care providers and deliver the anticipated benefits. We have analysed—and found issue with—the notion that a market in the NHS may be conceptually flawed (Chapter 5), and have begun to explore an alternative explanation: that the 'market' for secondary care is not working because it is being distorted and/or stifled; that, in effect, there exist so many barriers to its operation that it is questionable whether a market fully exists. In this section we build on the discussion of the previous—where the focus was on distortions in the market—by considering a further possibility: that the market, in addition, has been largely ineffective because it is being stifled—either intentionally or unintentionally. The section is divided into three parts: practical obstacles to tendering; underdeveloped skills in purchasers and providers; and the political and cultural environment. We then discuss these findings.

6B.1. Practical obstacles to tendering

A core mechanism to apply competitive pressure on secondary care providers within the market in the NHS (excluding elective services, where patients have a direct choice of provider) is the ability of PCTs to, where necessary, shift services around—to reward good service, punish bad and search for new ways of providing care. This requires tendering. However, in the course of the interviews PCT executives described numerous obstacles to putting services out to tender; the vast majority of which were corroborated by providers. In this section we present these in turn: a lack of alternative options; time-consuming tendering processes; bullying from acute trusts; poor quality of data; and a feeling of being locked into existing relationships.

a. Lack of alternative options

Although some interviewees felt that PCTs' theoretical ability to switch providers was alone enough to spur change in provider behaviour, generally, for the threat to be considered real, options must be available in the form of alternative providers. However, PCT executives—in our sample heath economy and validation sites—described a number of difficulties in finding both alternative NHS providers and potential providers in the private and voluntary sectors.

NHS providers

Participants frequently referred to two core difficulties in identifying alternative NHS providers. First, that NHS providers do not operate with excess capacity (or at least claim they do not[v]) and typically say they are 'full'. A PCT executive in one of our validation sites explained the implications of this for the success of the market:

> The problem is when we say [to x acute trust] we want to send you some more work, [they] say they don't think they can handle it and [the original acute trust] says they don't mind us switching because they're seeing rising numbers of patients anyway.

Provider executives tended to concur. One said: 'We work hard [here] to make sure we are not inviting demand; we don't want to have excess demand for services.' Another joked: 'We have to plead with PCTs to turn off the tap, so to speak.'

The second point is that because NHS providers reported operating at 'full' capacity, provider executives often said they felt little need to make any changes or service improvements in order to compete for business. 'We don't need to compete, we're as full as can be', said one. Others linked this to the fact that NHS funding has increased dramatically over the past decade, enabling providers to soak up latent demand. A provider executive reported:

> We're not sitting here thinking 'oh my word we're struggling with [maintaining] levels of activity', quite the opposite... simply being the local NHS provider has resulted in increasing demand over the past few years. We have not needed to take any other action.

Another reflected:

> It is still an expanding market. Only with the impact of the recession might we have to compete for commissioned services [in coming years].

Private and voluntary sector providers

The lack of options for PCTs in the private and voluntary sectors is explained by slightly different reasons. While some executives disputed that a lack of available providers was an issue (one PCT executive said, 'we've never had a problem... providers will usually emerge once they

---

[v] We say this because a number of PCT executives—and provider executives—felt providers could do more through improved efficiency, even when they reported being 'full'. Capacity can be measured in many ways, for example as maximum throughput given the current operations of a provider, or as potential throughput if the provider were operating at industry standards (or the level of the best standards).

know what we're after'), for others it was a genuine concern. One PCT executive reflected on particular problems in commissioning from the voluntary sector:

> It would be great to have a third sector provider of post-natal support services, but these initiatives tend to be run by three to five people, and the viability of such organisations is often lacking.

Another said, 'With some services there is just very little interest from the wider market', adding that responses to a recent tender for GP services had come from 'very flaky companies'. By way of explanation for this, interviewees drew attention to three issues: high bid costs; services being too small in nature for providers to take advantage of economies of scale; and cost disadvantages suffered by the private and voluntary sectors when compared with NHS providers (see section 6A.2). One PCT executive opined:

> [When commissioning services] we are often faced with a limited choice between NHS organisations that are able to take advantage of existing overheads.

b. Time consuming tendering processes

In making the decision to tender, and again in the act of tendering, PCTs must follow guidance set out in the *PCT Procurement Guide for Health Services* (see Annex A for a full explanation of what this entails).[8][vi] Once a provider has been chosen, in most circumstances PCTs must then use the appropriate NHS Standard Contract.

While DH and SHA officials we spoke with as part of this study did not feel the process was unnecessarily onerous—'I don't buy the argument that it's too complicated', one said—this was not the view of the majority of interviewees at PCTs and providers (NHS and non-NHS). Most considered the level of bureaucracy required in putting services out to tender to be 'long-winded' and out of proportion with the need to ensure transparency and taxpayer value for money. Some also drew attention to the additional impact of regulatory pressures such as the World Class Commissioning regime, which requires time

---

vi This is a 33 page document. The recommended strategy can be found in Annex A. It states procurement should adhere to four core principles: transparency; equality of treatment; non-discrimination; and proportionality.

and resources be put into proving that tendering has been done properly and, in the words of one executive, that 'all boxes have been ticked'. One private provider executive reported:

> EU public procurement regulations [under which much PCT commissioning operates] create a level of bureaucratic process, but this hasn't changed substantially in the last seven years. In my view the bureaucratic reaction of the NHS has changed enormously. I'm not sure whether it is just that in 2003 people weren't doing things by the book, but to me the thrust of World Class Commissioning seems to have created an end in itself.

A few participants felt in particular that some PCTs had become so consumed with the process of tendering that they had lost sight of the end goal of securing a better service for patients.

An additional concern, expressed particularly by PCT executives, was the threat of legal challenge from unsuccessful NHS bidders. One PCT executive explained:

> Over the past two years, there has been a massive increase in the number of legal challenges from providers that we have had to deal with. That is where the process becomes overly time consuming. If hospitals have not been successful with a bid, they think, 'why should I not challenge?'

The net result of the time and effort required to tender, according to some participants, was to stifle the motivation of PCTs to use the market. One PCT executive reported:

> Often when we see we need to commission a new service, we need that service in one to three months—not after the nine or so it can take to carry out and award a tendered contract. It is easier to contract with an existing provider.

A private provider executive agreed:

> The current tendering process is highly expensive and time-consuming, and I am sure that influences what seems like an instinct for PCTs to contract with current providers.

c. Bullying from NHS trusts

One of the more frequently cited obstacles to tendering was pushback, or bullying, from NHS (foundation) trusts. PCT executives reported many forms of this, such as trusts: claiming tenders undermined their plans for development; threatening to disengage with PCT initiatives or make work difficult for the PCTs in other ways; and threatening legal challenge as referred to above. One PCT executive said:

There is definitely the resolve [to tender services here] at the executive level... but when we try to put larger contracts out to tender, the NHS providers shout out that we are undermining their long-term work.

For providers in our sample health economy, this extended to colluding in opposition to PCT programmes. In response to national and regional schemes involving independent providers, for example, acute trusts initially refused to let their consultants work with such centres, and for such centres, out of hours.

The feelings of PCT executives were corroborated by provider executives, who seemed aware of the impact of their activity on PCTs. One reported:

I can see how competitive tendering could possibly bring some [of the] expected market benefits if it were carried out as intended, but it would depend on PCTs being strong, not weak. PCTs currently tend to hold back from competitive tendering and seem afraid to give business to one side or the other, as though they are intimidated by providers.

Another went further, commenting:

PCTs are scared of the providers' political power. They are afraid of putting services out to tender and angering the hospital providers. They are afraid that the hospitals will then go and do something to retaliate that will cause the PCT managers to lose their jobs.

d. Quality of data questionable

In interviews, PCT executives often referred to the importance of credible, complete data in order to: assess the performance of providers; decide which levers to use in driving performance and whether or not to tender; and to make effective judgements on the respective quality of bids received. However, most participants felt that although available data was improving, the current standard of data on provider quality, operational efficiency, and cost was not good enough. One reported:

Assessment of quality is not easy. There is not much published, and what is available is questionable and not always easy to compare [with data from other providers].

An IT expert familiar with the collection of data in our sample health economy said:

Quality of data is extremely poor... trusts have base IT administrative systems, but they don't often equate to what's going on. There is much duplication; and records are incomplete and held in unconnected systems that require armies of people to correct.

Looking specifically at data on costs, two provider executives, for example, could not name their most profitable services. One said:

> It's not surgical activity, because we are not efficient in theatre. It's more at the outpatient and diagnostic end of the spectrum. I'd probably say anti-coagulation services; we have very high throughput here, and it's cheap to deliver.

The implications of PCT executives not having full information on such matters are significant. One former DH official reported on the ease with which this means NHS organisations can pursue predatory pricing (illegal in other industries) without a PCT's knowledge, thereby distorting tenders in their favour:

> Many NHS providers will shift their overhead costs around to remove cost from services where they want to win competitive contracts, downloading them onto others where there is no competition.

e. PCTs feel locked into relationships with providers
Pulling the themes of this section together, obstacles to tendering were such that PCTs in our sample health economy—consistent with at least one of our validation sites—felt locked into existing relationships with acute trusts. One PCT executive reflected:

> Most of why we commission primarily from [the local acute trust] has to do with the inertia of the system. We have historically commissioned from them, and there is not much capacity elsewhere for us to be able to change providers if we wanted to.

Provider executives at acute trusts tended to assume similar relationships, repeatedly making references to 'the PCT' as opposed to differentiating between PCTs in the wider area that they could potentially gain business from.

6B.2. Underdeveloped skills on the part of purchasers and providers

Two participants in our study drew particular attention to the stifling effect that a lack of capability and skills can have on the effectiveness of a market. One focused on the purchasing side (and the role of PCTs in particular):

If you don't have commissioners who can make markets, administer failure [i.e. decommission services that are not delivering quality and value] and switch services away from failing providers, the market won't work. Period.

Another focused on the provider side:

[The market] is a necessary but not sufficient condition to drive improvement. It is not sufficient because organisations have to be capable of responding to competitive forces.

Our findings support these sentiments and suggest requisite skills are weak on both the purchasing and provision sides of the NHS market. Here, we present these weaknesses, beginning first with PCTs and then moving onto providers.

PCTs

We found the (internal) weakness of PCTs to stem from two related problems: weak management and underdeveloped commissioning skills, exemplified by an inability to follow through stated plans.

a. Weak management

Among our interviewees, including PCT executives, there was a wide-spread agreement that—with a few notable exceptions—management at PCTs tends to be weak, or at least weaker than in acute trusts. One PCT executive reflected:

There is [an] issue with the quality of managers at PCTs, though I hope we would be an exception!

Another, who had previously worked in the private sector, said:

Decision-making is very diffuse in that it takes so long to affect anything that in the private sector would be decided around the board table after submissions.

A private provider executive reported:

The calibre of people [at PCTs] is a problem... most are not commercially focused. PCTs rely too much on consultancy fees paid to unimpressive people who are constantly changing. There's no continuity.

Many participants reflected on the underlying reasons for these weaknesses. Some considered it to be because PCTs are relatively new organisations formed from community care providers, and subsequently are often led by managers whose background is in provision, not commissioning. As one provider executive put it, 'everyone's trying to learn from pretty much a zero base of under-standing'. Others linked it to a confusing policy environment (see section 5.3). Others still, felt it was because top managers are attracted to supply side jobs. Generally, interviewees felt executive positions at acute trusts often come with: higher pay; more freedom and control over internal processes; greater prestige due to the public's perception of hospitals as cornerstones of the NHS; and potentially more job security. One provider executive put this in stark terms: 'Acute trusts are where the action is.'

b. Underdeveloped commissioning skills

Consistent with there being weak management, we also found PCTs to be underdeveloped as *commissioning* organisations, in many cases lacking even basic commissioning skills. One provider executive reflected:

> I really do not think PCTs have the requisite skills. Even with World Class Commissioning, skills are weak. They are still not commissioning well even at a basic level—forget world class.

Three particular skill areas seem underdeveloped: strategy and decision-making; performance management; and tendering. Addition-ally, and within all of these, we found there to be a lack of clinical input.

Strategy and decision-making

Throughout the course of the interviews we were presented with numerous examples of poor planning and decision-making. One provider executive commented:

> [PCTs] are very good at the philosophical part [of commissioning], but the strategy and implementation are lacking. Simple things, like not having enough rooms or offices to carry out a service, are often overlooked.

An SHA executive commented on a tendency for PCTs to follow policy guidance without forming a coherent strategy themselves:

> Commissioning was meant to be a strategic tool [but] there's too much mindless commissioning, which is no better than mindlessly carrying on as we always have done.

'We have to be more subtle in contracting', a PCT executive added.

In our sample health economy, the inability to plan and take forward decisions manifested itself particularly in a failure on the part of PCTs to follow through strategies to move services out of hospitals and into the community. Nearly every provider executive we spoke to mentioned this issue. One explained:

> PCTs... advocate 'de-hospitalising' services while at the same time continuing to commission community and other services from our hospitals... Each year they tell us what they plan to purchase, but then what they actually purchase is much different.

Another said:

> The PCT planned to remove services from the hospital and create an outpatient facility instead, which we agreed to, but then when we went to move our patients, the facility was not ready.

More generally, PCTs found it difficult to integrate decision-making processes across various spectrums of care. One PCT executive reflected on this:

> [It is difficult]... perhaps it is the sense of instability that would ensue—once we transform one service, we will have to put such changes into effect throughout the PCT.

Performance management

The general picture we obtained of weakness in PCTs' performance management of providers is reflected in two related issues.[vii] The first concerns the tendency of PCTs to micro-manage contracts. One participant argued:

> PCTs have been managing the status quo rather than driving change, preferring ludicrous performance management routes than looking for alternative options.

A private provider executive said:

> The way [PCTs] police contracts sometimes verges on being Kafkaesque. There's a profound unwillingness to allow the independent sector to have any flexibility, which in my view is a mistake... In the private sector, there is a lot more give and take, which is mutually beneficial as it incentivises suppliers to be flexible.

---

vii We say general, because we did see some examples of good practice such as that reported later in this subsection.

The second issue concerns PCTs' broader lack of attention to managing relationships with providers (see Annex B for a fuller discussion of different approaches to tendering and contracting across the industry). Some PCTs were forthright about this and were attempting to tackle it. One executive, in one of our validation sites, reported:

> I think a lot of the push-back and underpowered-PCT sentiment is settled with relationship management. Maybe our tools as PCTs are not based on policy levers, but on being firm, having the right information, and on intellectual power.

She continued:

> When things are contentious I invite [the chairman of the hospital trust] over for tea and we discuss them. You can have tough negotiations and still go out and have a drink afterwards. The NHS doesn't seem to understand this. Private sector purchasers have very good relationships with their suppliers.

Another PCT executive, in our sample health economy, reported:

> We are developing partnerships between buyers and sellers of care... that is the way it is done in other industries.

Another said:

> [A constructive relationship] allows the supplier to shape services to meet our needs because they know the services will be purchased.

However, this was not the norm. One PCT executive reflected:

> Clinicians should hold the pen on specification and service design, with us holding the ring on whether it is appropriate to the outcome we wish to achieve... [but] this does not always happen because relationships aren't always great.

A private provider executive reported:

> There's no sense of collaboration, rather [PCTs], mirroring attitudes in the DH, see their remit as being to police, which doesn't bring value for money.

Another provider, referring to the opening of a new facility, reported how a PCT executive had introduced himself with the words: 'Hi, I'm x, from the PCT. I'm the one who's supposed to be hitting you.'

Tendering

In this sub-section we are concerned with a PCT's strategic decision to tender and the management of the aspects of the tendering process that are within the PCT's control (i.e. not including structural concerns about the tendering process *outside* a PCT's control, see section 6B.1b).

Looking first at the decision to tender, referred to above, many participants felt PCTs decided to tender less out of a strategic desire to actively look for better, alternative, services, and more as a means of exerting control over existing providers or to be seen to be doing the 'right thing' under the World Class Commissioning framework. One PCT executive reported:

> This system of encouraging everything to be put out to tender [even where services are of good quality] has resulted in a lot of failed services and adversarial relationships.

In addition, participants felt that PCTs (in general) did not have sufficient understanding that different services may require different approaches to tendering, or that in some situations tendering may not be appropriate at all. One PCT executive argued:

> I believe PCTs should have long-term, core contracts with the NHS providers, perhaps even up to 10 years, with the providers knowing very well that smaller, related, services may be put out to tender.

A private provider executive said:

> Although prudent organisations might have a look around, if it's some of the best why not just say 'I'm happy with this, let's continue.'

Turning now to management of the tendering process itself, we found many examples of poor practice, including: badly written tenders; poor engagement with bidders on the nature of the service tendered for; and failures to follow tenders through. One provider executive reported:

> [The PCT] has asked us again and again to tender for services that we have historically provided... and we do. But then nothing seems to happen. We are never sure what is going on.

Another commented:

> Often the contract [tendered for] isn't awarded, or even re-negotiated with us, and we all go back to the existing provision contract.

Procurement regulations exist, but we found such regulations typically to be poorly understood, inconsistently applied and applied with too narrow constraint by a majority of PCTs. We found certain

PCTs, for example, to be using contracts of over 160 pages for community services' contracts worth little more than £70,000 per annum (i.e. below the threshold for tender).

Providers

In this sub-section we focus attention on capability in the supply side of the market, in NHS providers. The critical point is that the majority of acute trusts (including FTs) we spoke to appeared either unprepared or ill-equipped to operate in a market and, in turn, to respond to the needs of commissioners and patients. Here, we present our findings relating to these deficiencies.

a. 'Classic monopolists'

Typically, we found unwillingness among acute trusts to engage with PCTs and PbC groups and to accept the authority of any purchasing organisation *per se*. There were exceptions. One provider executive said:

> We certainly don't agree on everything with [the PCT], but we have shared values. We trust them, and we work together.

However, in general, we found provider executives sought to carry on with their own agendas, regardless of PCTs and the market. One interviewee put it as such:

> Typically [acute trusts] are classic monopolists and hate it when someone invades their turf.

We have already cited examples of bullying (see section 6B.1c) but, more commonly, provider executives referred to PCTs with a degree of disdain. One said:

> More things happen at a PCT's say-so than would have done before, and should do. They wield the false threat that they can take business elsewhere.

Others appeared set on making things as difficult for PCTs as possible. One PCT executive, for example, described an incident where '[an FT] told their clinicians that on no account should they engage with our PbC groups', effectively blocking attempts at quality improvement. Another exclaimed:

> [Acute trusts] are addicted to tweaking the game in their favour and are often actually downright rude.

b. Cost control in NHS providers

We also found many acute trusts, for the most part, to be ill-equipped to operate in a market, primarily because they do not understand their costs and/or do not have systems in place to utilise cost data effectively (including some FTs). One SHA executive emphasised the significance of this point:

> The issue of provider economics is very important. Not least because if any PCT does pull 20 per cent or so of a provider's business away into the community, acute trusts will fall over if they don't understand their cost base.

On the first point—understanding costs—we found varying levels of competence. At the level of the best, one provider executive said 'we can produce a hospital bill per patient, down to individual Health Resource Groups (HRGs)'.[viii] Another asserted:

> I would be pretty confident that a clinician will know how much he/she earns the trust and how much x procedure they do costs... every consultant and clinical programme group is assessed on the basis of patient satisfaction, financial service line management and clinical outcomes.

However, at the level of the worst, one provider executive said:

> We still have functional budgets, with little cross-charging. Some departments therefore appear to have healthy surpluses, but it's often because they don't cover overhead costs.

More common was for financial understanding to be centralised in finance departments, with little awareness at clinical, departmental or ward-level.

On the second point—actually using cost data—most did not apparently use data on costs in any systematic way to drive quality and efficiency. One provider executive reported:

> I am convinced that we remain grossly inefficient and spend a lot of time managing processes which could be improved. If we were to have better systems and processes we would have excess capacity, and we could release this into the system to either develop and improve services further or ultimately reduce the level of health spend.

A medically-qualified executive said:

---

viii Healthcare Resource Groups (HRGs) provide a means of categorising the treatment of patients in order to monitor and evaluate the use of resources.

> We don't monitor costs on a daily basis. We are reliant on others telling us, based on theatre time, bed days, cost of prosthesis etc....

Others seemed to conceptualise efforts to improve cost awareness as more of a one-off, rather than an ongoing, process. One medically-qualified participant explained:

> We had meetings with the surgeons, got a financial breakdown of what we needed to do to improve—for example, looking at profit-loss vis-à-vis what happens in the private sector... We've got to the point now where we've stopped asking for them, because we're turning profit.

And others, too, argued that productivity improvement is, in any case, impossible. '[The cost of prosthesis] is perhaps the only thing we can have an effect on', one medically-qualified executive said. 'NHS services are working at full tilt. So if the inference is we can see more [patients], we must be adversely affecting quality.'

6B.3. Stifling political and cultural environment

At this juncture it is worth referring back to section 5.3, where we considered findings in support of the thesis that the market in the NHS might be flawed because it will forever be quashed by the political and centralised nature of the organisation. Although we cast doubt on the extent to which this argument is true, our findings on the impact of: constantly changing policy; government targets; and reluctance to countenance hospital closures, almost certainly *stifle* the market and should be kept in mind here. In this section we add to them by focusing on participants' comments concerning the culture of the NHS. Specifically, we found the market to be stifled by: continued 'command and control' attitudes; an attachment to the 'comfortable life'; reluctance on the part of providers to consider patients as consumers and patients to consider themselves as such; and the promulgation of the 'NHS family'.

a. Command and control

Here, we are concerned with the comments of participants with regard to the legacy of the NHS as a centralised system driven by the 'command and control' of government. We uncovered two primary concerns. First, a large number of participants felt many people working in the NHS are ideologically opposed to any pretence of a market (including some participants themselves, both PCT and provider executives). One PCT participant said, for example, '[There are many who] feel the inclusion of the private sector in any form within the NHS is ethically wrong.' A private provider added 'I have actually had a PCT chief executive say to me: "I don't believe in competition".'

A DH official described the implications of this sentiment:

Most people in most places have tried to block [the market]; and, where private providers have been used, it is typically for short-term goals... not strategically.

The second concern is that even where no ideological opposition to the idea of a market exists, there are many who have worked in the NHS all their lives and are used to working in a 'command and control' environment. One PCT executive reflected:

I do think that many current managers were trained in a command and control system, and for policy to now be pushing competition—it's a forced culture change. Of course there are going to be some people who will resist.

A provider executive, from one of our validation sites, concurred:

Competitive forces are not comfortable for us brought up in a monopoly world, which hasn't served patients well enough.

Another provided an example of the changes required:

Too many process are still designed around targets and workforce restrictions, rather than looking at processes first in light of patient need.

b. An attachment to the 'comfortable life'

Related to the question of change is a sense conveyed by participants— provider executives in particular—that the monopoly structure of the NHS, isolated from market pressure, has traditionally permitted a comfortable life (if not for CEOs, then for those further down organisations) that is proving hard for the market to shift. Two interviewees, for example, described experiences of managing consultants who operated very differently when working in the private sector, as opposed to within the NHS. One medically-qualified executive commented:

It's a question of having the will. Four surgeons didn't turn up for work here yesterday, blaming the snow. In the private sector they'd all turn up... In the health service there just isn't the will to work too hard, because you won't get fired and you've got your pension. We need to embrace the idea that more work equals more security. You can't get rid of those who are just here to get a pension... Just don't have that bacon butty that makes you late for starting your list.

Along similar lines, a private provider executive revealed:

I know for a fact that a surgeon in an unnamed NHS trust takes 2½ hours to do a hip replacement that he does in 45 minutes at [one of our hospitals]. Management struggles to deal with this because the surgeon can play the clinical card. Maybe we should have PbR for surgeons?

Others focused on the difficulty of asking GPs to change their behaviour, thereby stifling the effects of competitive tendering. One PCT executive commented:

The majority of GPs still use traditional pathways... [the independent sector-run diagnostics service] was supposed to move services out of the hospital, but GPs are not referring to them.

Another said:

[When PCTs] go out to tender, GPs will say they're on board [but] just want to carry on as before.

A few participants also criticised PbC groups (and PCTs) for being 'too protective' of their assets and of paying 'over-the-odds' to keep services in-house. One PCT executive reflected,

Generally, things that already exist are hard to change or de-commission... the NHS has a huge inertia in maintaining the status quo.

c. Reluctant consumers

There are two points to note on the notion of patients as 'consumers' in the NHS market. The first is that patients have, thus far, proved reluctant to take on this role. The second is that providers have been reluctant to consider them as such.

On the first point—and while this study did not involve speaking to patients directly—most PbC and PCT executives said it was common for patients in our sample health economy to say to their GPs, 'you choose', when presented a with a choice of provider for elective care. Reflecting on the data they had available, participants reported that only a small percentage of patients actually research the quality of care at hospitals and make decisions on where to be treated. Most patients, one participant said, 'tend to think the best care is by nature provided in hospital'. Provider executives, for their part, tended to refer to patient surveys that either they or local trusts had carried out affirming patient preference for their local hospital. One said:

> Year after year we carry out consultations asking what local patients want, where they want to go, and they always want to be sent to their local DGH, except in the case of cancer or other specialist services. I think this is similar throughout England.[ix]

On the second point, we also found that acute trusts, by and large, had not embraced the notion of patients as 'consumers' or 'customers'. One provider executive reflected:

> There is a sense in which the system does not want to open up to 'patient power'. NHS staff don't like the word 'customer'.

Another went so far as to say 'no-one wants to go to a private hospital when they're sick'. Others, too, reflected on the reluctance of GPs to offer choice. One PCT executive commented: 'GPs are not very receptive to the idea of referring patients elsewhere.'

d. The 'NHS family'

Binding together all the findings presented in this section is the impact on the market of a wider, deep-seated cultural reverence for something that is 'the NHS'. This was frequently described as a powerful influence on actions. One interviewee reflected:

> I do think many people in the UK—DH and NHS employees included—were brought up to behold the NHS as something culturally significant, almost infallible. And I think that these concepts stay with people and may come out in unexpected ways, even when logically they know otherwise.

A provider executive explained how he thought this tends to stifle the market:

> [There is] a fundamental problem in current market policy: the DH promotes competition and devotes substantial resources to its implementation, yet it also advocates the cultural sanctity and historic importance of the NHS... I do not

---

ix This can be disputed. In November 2009, for example, 26,733 patients across England chose to go to independent sector providers at the point of referral using Choose and Book (Moore, A., 'More patients pick private care', *HSJ*, 4 February 2010).

believe many people have bought into the idea that the NHS is the organisation that procures health care for the public and where that health care is delivered should not matter.

We found two aspects of this cultural sanctity to provide particularly powerful breaks on the market. First, there seems to be a reluctance on the part of PCTs to look outside 'the NHS family' in deciding on providers—either out of reverence for the NHS, or for fear of political consequences. This did not hold universally. One PCT executive, in one of the validation sites, stated:

Speaking personally, it should always be about quality and value, irrespective of the source that drives it.

However, he went on to reflect that:

There is still a culture of supporting the local NHS provider to the extent some PCTs are reluctant to transfer services out.

Another PCT executive from a different validation site argued:

I do think PCTs need to have the courage to do what's right, even in the face of political resistance. Recently, we pushed ahead and opened a privately-run 'Darzi Centre' against local GP wishes, because we knew it would be best for patients. So far patients love it and ask to go there. We also closed a community hospital about a year and a half ago. There was resistance to that too, although mostly from the existing staff (and their unions).

Some felt the same cultural sentiment also prevented NHS providers from actively competing with each other. One interviewee explained:

It is culturally difficult, given that the NHS has been seen as a single organisation for so long, to now see other NHS organisations as competitors. Foundation trusts are susceptible to being blackmailed into not competing by the 'NHS family'.

A provider executive in our sample health economy, for example, said: 'we have never gone in with an intention to take business away from others'.

The second aspect of concern in relation to the NHS family is that it encourages a 'them *versus* us' attitude between the NHS and voluntary/private sector providers, rather than seeing the latter as potential partners in the drive to achieve better health care. Again, this did not hold universally. One PCT executive said: 'We need both the NHS and the private sector to work together.' However, more than a few participants expressed contempt for independent sector involvement. One PCT executive said:

> There is a general suspicion of anything tied to the private sector among GPs and patients alike.

A provider executive, despite later acknowledging the independent sector's part in achieving the 18-week referral-to-treatment target, put it in more blunt terms:

> As a concept, I think [use of the private sector] stinks. [Meeting the 18-week target] has been wonderful for the system as a whole, but I think we should now try to implement this within our own NHS.

Another said:

> As I have got older and more experienced, I've become more and more suspicious of private care... You know, the consultants at the ISTC are from Eastern Europe or South Africa; they have not been trained in the NHS.

One private provider reported how, when his company was commissioned to provide care for the NHS, 'NHS doctors ignored the private healthcare clinic staff at local meetings, barred them from training courses, and made it extremely difficult for them to integrate into the medical community, which may have an adverse effect on quality of care.' He continued: 'Some NHS physicians walk out of the room when they enter.'

Another participant reflected:

> It is strange because the majority of private care in the UK is purchased by these very providers [NHS trusts] in order to meet their targets... and also, because GPs are private providers themselves, employed by the practice.

6B.4. Discussion

In the latter part of this report we have considered in some detail what lies behind our core finding: that the market in the NHS, by and large, has thus far failed to 1) have the intended impact on the behaviour of secondary care providers, and 2) drive the expected benefits— improved quality, efficiency, innovation, responsiveness to customers, and equity—on any meaningful or systematic scale.

Initially (Chapter 5), we presented evidence to support the viewpoint that there may be something inherently flawed with the concept of a market in the NHS. However, while pointing to a need for reform in certain areas, this account did not seem to fully explain why the market, on the whole, has thus far failed to deliver—not least because we did not see enough evidence that a market is truly operational for such a conclusion to be drawn. We followed this discussion (in section 6A) by presenting evidence that the market may instead have been ineffective because it is being distorted in fundamental ways, not least due to a structural imbalance inhibiting the ability of purchasers (patients, PCTs and practice-based commissioners) to effectively influence providers and significant obstacles to real diversity in supply due to the lack of a level playing field between NHS and non-NHS providers. In this section (6B) we have focused on additional barriers that have tended to stifle the market—a combination of practical obstacles to tendering, underdeveloped skills on the part of purchasers and providers, and an oppressive political and cultural environment. Combined with the flaws found in the idea that the market is flawed, it can be argued that these barriers alone explain a large part of why anticipated behaviours and benefits from the market thus far have failed to materialise. This is consistent with other studies,[x] not least simulations conducted by The King's Fund which indicate the default response of the NHS is likely to be a rejection of the market and competition.[9]

Indeed, the single largest factor inhibiting the success of the market is almost certainly the prevailing culture of the NHS, which is encapsulated in the dual legacy of 'command and control' and the emotive notion of the 'NHS family'. Ingrained in many staff working in

---

[x] Looking at the skills of PCTs, for example, in the Audit Commission's use of resources assessment of PCTs in 2008/09 just 53 per cent scored above minimum standards for 'managing finances'; 28 per cent for 'governing the business'; and 16 per cent for 'managing resources'. Not one PCT scored a level 4 rating ('significantly exceeds minimum requirements') for any category. Audit Commission, *Auditors Local Evaluation and Use of Resources 2008/09: Summary Results for NHS trusts and primary care trusts,* London: Audit Commission, 2009. On the provider side, as at January 2010 only 52 per cent (89 out of 169) of acute (non-mental health) trusts nationally had reached sufficient levels of financial control to gain FT status; a status that was intended to become a minimum standard. http://www.monitor-nhsft.gov.uk/

the NHS and promulgated by the politicians,[xi] the cultural sanctity of the NHS alone can explain many of the most intractable problems with the market: why acute trusts hold so much political power; why the inclination of PCTs is to micro-manage contracts and pursue adversarial relationships with providers, rather than working with them; why there are pressures to leave such a bureaucratic trail when tendering (in case a service ends up going outside the 'family'); why independent sector provision has reached nothing like the 15 per cent of elective care initially envisaged by the Labour Government under Tony Blair;[10(xii)] and, ultimately, why other approaches driving performance have thus far been more effective than the market itself.

---

xi For example, in the first 2010 televised election debate, Conservative Party leader, David Cameron, said 'I think the NHS is a wonderful, wonderful thing... I went from hospital to hospital... and the sense of vocation and love you get from people who work in the NHS makes me incredibly proud of this country. I think it is special.'

xii In 2008, Laing & Buisson estimated the figure to be just 3.6 per cent.

What should be done?

It is worth returning to the original aims of our study, which were to shed light on: whether the market for secondary care in the NHS, as currently configured, is an effective means for driving performance, and in turn whether the market offers a solution to the NHS's productivity imperative. Ultimately, our reasoning was this:

1. The financial challenge facing the NHS is unprecedented, with five years of near-static growth in funding ahead. In order to do little more than maintain existing standards of care (in the face of inflation and rising demand), it is estimated that the NHS will have to achieve productivity improvements of around four to six per cent *year-on-year*.[1] This is higher than the average annual increase across private sector industry over the past decade;

2. The experience of other industries, including some public services, suggests that markets (when placed within a proper and appropriate regulatory framework) have succeeded in driving such productivity while also improving quality and stimulating innovation;[2]

3. The very reason for introducing a market into the NHS was to attempt to harness such benefits (efficiency, quality and innovation), given the perceived failure of past reliance on central direction and/or professionalism;[i]

4. However, whether the market is delivering such benefits or not is something of an elusive question. Despite an increasing number of academic studies on various aspects of the market, conclusions

---

[i] Evidence suggests central direction may achieve results in areas specifically targeted, but tends to lead to a risk-averse, culture of compliance where that which is not targeted risks falling to comparative neglect. The values held by those working in the NHS have driven many to innovate and centre care processes on the needs and wants of patients, but also has been used to put professional needs and research interests first.

have tended to be somewhat ambiguous.[ii] Political support for the idea of a market is also waning, and many politicians and staff alike are asking whether we can afford a market in the tight financial times ahead (making the consequences of failure greater).

Against such a backdrop, we set the goal of providing further insight into just how effective the market has been. To do so, we focused on secondary care—where the market is most embedded in the NHS—and asked the following questions:

a. Is the market—for contracts with PCTs and, in the case of electives, directly for patients—having its intended impact on the behaviour of secondary care providers?

b. And, if so, is that behaviour bringing about the expected benefits—defined as improved quality, efficiency, innovation, responsiveness to customers, and equity?[iii]

In adopting a largely qualitative approach using semi-structured interviews, we also endeavoured to gauge *why* the market is working (or not), in order to inform policymakers of future options for the NHS.

We recognise the limitations of this approach. Qualitative work cannot fully answer the question: 'Does the market work?'—not least because of response bias (i.e. people painting a better picture of their achievements than is the case). Moreover, in focusing on one health economy, our findings may say more about experiences and relationships in one particular area than about the impact of the market in the NHS across England. Given further time, we would ideally also have sought additional input from frontline clinicians and patients. However, we did seek to minimise such limitations by cross-comparing each participant's view with others in the same organisation and nearby organisations; and by validating our findings through seeking the opinions of those in other health economies. Our contribution to the

---

ii The DH-funded Health Reforms Evaluation Programme, coordinated by Nicholas Mays at the London School of Hygiene and Tropical Medicine, has looked at five aspects of the market reforms and will be reporting in 2010. Other major centres of research in this area include the London School of Economics under Julian Le Grand, and The King's Fund.

iii A full account of our methodology can be found in Chapter 3.

debate is to assemble and analyse the thoughts and opinions of people across the different purchaser and provider organisations that currently make up the NHS market, and to provide in-depth insight into how the market is operating on the ground, how successful it has been and why.

In direct answer to our research question(s), what emerged quite clearly from our findings is that, by and large, the market in the NHS is yet to 1) have the intended impact on the behaviour of secondary care providers and 2) drive the expected benefits—improved quality, efficiency, innovation, responsiveness to customers, and equity—on any meaningful or systematic scale. This was the impression developed from both our sample health economy and—if to a slightly lesser extent—our validation sites. There are isolated and subtle examples of the market having the anticipated benefits: greater customer-focus; increased image-consciousness; increased awareness of the actions of other organisations; providers made to 'think' when tenders are put out; and providers, in more than a few cases, using the threat of losing business—even if more hypothetical than real—to motivate change internally. Organisations have also been forced to look harder at their efficiency. However, such effects are far from the widespread benefits and changes in behaviour hoped for by protagonists of the NHS market. In particular, it is clear that there are many other factors that drive behaviour and performance in secondary care organisations. Though it is not possible to measure the relative importance of any one factor to any degree of certainty, most executives we spoke to felt factors such as targets, a desire to achieve high CQC ratings, a culture of continuous quality improvement, and professional pride have had far greater impact on driving performance than has the market. This is consistent with the findings of the majority of academic studies on the market in the NHS to date, including the most recent by The King's Fund on patient choice.[3]

The question we then focused on is *why* the market has not, for the most part, been much of a success; a question that has profound implications for the future of health policy in England, in the tight financial climate. We found the issues described by participants— executives and clinicians at PCTs, NHS trusts, foundation trusts and practice-based commissioning groups—to point to two possible scenarios:

1. The concept of a market operating in the NHS is flawed and therefore any attempt to introduce one is unlikely to be effective;

2. A market can be effective in the NHS, but it is not currently working because it is being distorted and/or stifled.

The first scenario deals with concerns—such as the existence of market failures and whether there is something in the political and centralised nature of the NHS that will forever quash market incentives—that should forever remain at the forefront of policymakers' minds. However, the idea that a market is conceptually flawed when applied within the NHS was ultimately dismissed because a) where the market has been used (i.e. where providers report feeling competitive pressure from patient choice and where PCTs have put services out to tender and chosen alternative providers) participants did report *some* examples of the positive effects anticipated. And, most importantly, b) we did not find enough evidence that a 'market' has truly been functioning within the NHS to date. Currently, too many barriers exist to the operation of such mechanisms that it seems incorrect to analyse or draw conclusions on their effectiveness. (Indeed, this in itself can explain some of the negative consequences of the market detailed by participants.[iv])

The second scenario—that the NHS market is largely failing to deliver because it is being distorted and stifled—we found more persuasive. Specifically, there appears to be: structural imbalance inhibiting the ability of purchasers (patients, PCTs and practice-based commissioners) to effectively influence providers; significant obstacles to *real* diversity in the supply side due to the lack of a level playing field between NHS and non-NHS providers; and adverse incentives stemming from payment-by-results and GP-led commissioning. Addressing these may well lead to a more effective market.

More significantly, the market is unquestionably being stifled. Important barriers include practical obstacles to tendering; underdeveloped skills on the part of both purchasers and providers; and an oppressive political and cultural environment. The strongest

---

iv For example, there is a case to be made that acute trusts have been able to dictate terms to PCTs and patients (their 'customers'), precisely because they do not see the threat of losing business as real.

factor here is almost certainly the latter; the prevailing culture of the NHS characterised by a legacy of 'command and control' and the emotive notion of the 'NHS family'. There is a fundamental dichotomy presented by politicians promulgating the cultural significance of the NHS—presenting it as something of an infallible system of hospital provision—while at the same time, advocating the need for a market to motivate innovation and improvements in efficiency and quality of care. Without wanting to repeat the discussion of section 6B, the cultural reverence for the NHS as a provider system (rather than as a system of universal health care coverage), alone can explain many of the most intractable problems with the market: why acute trusts hold so much political power; why the inclination of PCTs is to micro-manage contracts; why there are pressures to leave such a bureaucratic trail when tendering (in case a service ends up going outside the 'family'); and why independent sector provision has reached nothing like the 15 per cent of elective care envisaged by the Labour Government under Tony Blair. [4(v)]

We believe these findings are significant. On balance, we consider the evidence presented here in support of the conclusion that the market in the NHS is largely failing to deliver because it is being stifled and distorted is *stronger* than the evidence supporting the case that it is failing to deliver because it is conceptually flawed. While care must forever be taken to preserve the values the NHS holds true (universal, comprehensive coverage, free-at-the-point-of-delivery), in no uncertain terms do we need to encourage the government to support and promote the NHS market as a means out of its financial crisis, and to seek to remove the barriers (not least ministerial influence itself) that are currently distorting and stifling it. We see the following as a model with which the full potential of the market in the NHS could be achieved:[(vi)]

- **Ministerial commitment to a market.** For the market to work, commissioners and providers above all need clarity and stability: a sustained commitment on behalf of the government to the market

---

[v] In 2008, Laing & Buisson estimated the figure to be just 3.6 per cent.

[vi] We recognise these recommendations possibly go further than what may be drawn from our study.

and to principles and parameters that support it (but which otherwise permit flexibility). These can be found in the *Principles and Rules for Cooperation and Competition* as originally formulated in the NHS Operating Framework 2008/09 (see Annex C).[5] The tendency (which shows no signs of abating) to change organisational structures on a scant evidence base, has been damaging enough in times of plenty; in times of severe financial strain the consequences could be far worse. [vii]

- **A new story for the NHS.** Promoting the cultural sanctity of the NHS as a system of hospital provision greater than the sum of its parts should end. Instead, politicians should tell a new story of the NHS that is truer to its founding principles: as a health service that supports civil society through providing high quality universal, collective, health care coverage, free-at-the-point-of-use, using the best providers available (NHS or non-NHS).

- **Ministerial and DH support for commissioners.** Ministerial support should be first and foremost for commissioners, not providers. The role of the DH needs to be recast, from considering itself the headquarters of a large corporation of providers, to being the 'headquarters' of a commissioning system, representing patients. One way of doing so could be to split the DH into a provider arm and a commissioning arm.

  o **The provider arm** would be a temporary structure, intended to ensure all secondary care providers that can become foundation trusts do so (regulated by Monitor), and all that cannot are subject to alternative solutions (taken over by other FTs or other independent providers, merged, reconfigured, or where unsustainable, closed).

  o **The commissioning arm**—which could form the remit of an independent commissioning board—would: ensure there is an environment conducive to effective commissioning; develop

---

vii It is hard to put a price on the cost to the NHS of constant changes to the system and constant ministerial interference, but as one participant noted, at the most basic level, 'it is difficult to make comparisons year on year'—which is crucial in commissioning and modern management.

commissioning skills; define what PCTs are expected to achieve; assess their performance; and institute an appropriate failure regime. It should be run by people who have experience of 'commissioning' (i.e. procurement) in health care, the NHS and other industries, and who are committed to supporting PCTs as impartial commissioners. If satisfied that a PCT has a rigorous business plan, this arm/board should offer public support where difficult decisions have to be made around re-configuration. It should not promote preference for any particular provider or type of provider (NHS or non-NHS).

Initial tasks should include:

- Developing a more effective and less 'tick-box'-type regulatory framework for PCTs;

- Encouraging a less burdensome and prescriptive approach to tendering;

- Encouraging 'relational' contracting (see Annex B);

- Simplifying standard NHS contracts to shorter forms tailored to contract value;

- Working towards a system of more integrated payment for non-elective care (i.e. the management of long-term conditions);

- Devising programmes to attract top managers to PCTs and developing commissioning skills;

- Encouraging PCTs to merge, or work collaboratively, where there is a sound case for doing so;

- Working towards local contracting of GPs.

- **The role of SHAs** could be re-cast as outposts of any commissioning arm of the DH.

- **PCTs should be framed along the lines of local health insurers,** as representatives of patients and the local population, charged with the goal of securing the best possible health care for them within a constrained budget. In doing so they should lose their 'primary/ community care' slant and should act as independent, unbiased, evaluators and purchasers free from institutional allegiance. PCTs should be directly engaged with patients and occupied in:

o **Effectively defining the needs of their populations** in terms of health indices, clinical outcomes, ease of access to services, and types of services;

o **Commissioning services that meet these needs and challenge those that do not;**

o **Horizon-scanning** for the latest and best technologies and service models (particularly 'disruptive'[viii] ones); and **bringing in new providers** to challenge the working practices of existing organisations;

o **Benchmarking providers to motivate improvements in performance and eliminate inefficiency,** challenging such things as referral patterns, outdated clinical models, and in-patient length of stay;

o Avoiding the temptation to tender prescriptively and resort to lengthy and cumbersome contracts, seeking instead to **embrace a model of 'relational' contracting** (see Annex B);

o Where appropriate, seeking to commission services across primary and secondary care.[ix]

- **Providers should be placed in a competitive market.** There are a number of structural and practical issues that should be addressed in order to reduce the primacy of acute trusts over the health system:

[viii] 'Disruptive' innovations enable things that could only previously be done expensively and by highly-skilled practitioners to be done at much lower cost by people who are less well-trained. An example in health care would be diabetics now being able to measure their HbA1C levels themselves.

[ix] We are not convinced by proposed moves to hand the majority of commissioning over to GPs. On the basis of this study, we would prefer a model where PCTs hold broad responsibility and seek to engage clinicians across the primary and secondary care spectrum.

o **The Collaboration and Competition Panel should operate on a statutory basis** in order to give it real 'teeth' and investigative powers;

o **Full cost allocation and accounting should be enforced.** This should form part of the remit for the CCP;

o **A level playing field** for the private and voluntary sectors should be created by ironing out cost disadvantages suffered by these sectors *vis-à-vis* the NHS (currently around 14 per cent). This applies particularly to pensions;

o **The publication of comparative data on quality and cost** should be advanced, preferably through multiple sources; and regulatory regimes—such as the CQC—should be streamlined across sectors. In addition, Monitor should encourage the expansion of cost awareness out of finance departments to clinical leads and beyond;

o **A proper failure regime for NHS providers, equivalent to going into administration in the private sector, should be instituted**, where assets can be disposed of, taken over or reconfigured according to their quality and viability.

We recognise this is a challenging agenda. We recognise, also, that there will be many who object to the conclusions we have drawn either on ideological grounds, or for fear of the consequences of market failure. The latter is a vital concern and must always be carefully considered. On the former, we wish to emphasis only this: that we recommend sustaining and supporting a regulated market in the NHS not out of any ideological commitment to markets, but based on the evidence found in this study and evidence contained in other recent research (to be clear, also, we are not talking about 'privatising' health care,[x] rather about using the market within a framework of universal coverage, free-at-the-point-of-use). We see a market in the NHS as the best course open to us, as a society, in order to secure high quality care for all in the tight financial times ahead. It will upset the status quo and

---

[x] The mainstay of the NHS, GPs, have been independently contracted businesses since 1948, for example.

will require real courage on behalf of all actors, but will also provide an open door to new ideas and new ways of doing things that the NHS will so desperately need in the coming years. After all, if a provider could offer a better service to the NHS for significantly less cost, would you, as a taxpaying citizen, ignore it?

Annex A

Department of Health guidance on PCT procurement and tendering

DH guidance on procurement for PCTs is found in the *PCT Procurement Guide for Health Services*,[1] a 33 page document. It states procurement should adhere to four core principles: transparency; equality of treatment; non-discrimination; and proportionality. In particular, it recommends that PCTs should 'adopt a procurement process that suits the nature of services being commissioned'.

There is flexibility for PCTs both in the decision to tender and the type of tender issued—be it single tender action (i.e. uncontested); open competition; restricted competition or competitive dialogue—and PCTs are encouraged to both horizon-scan for potential options and engage providers in long-term strategic partnerships.

The concern expressed in this study over the bureaucracy involved in procurement stems less from the overall framework prescribed by the *Procurement Guide*, but by its small print. This is particularly so when the *Procurement Guide* is placed alongside other rules, regulations and guidance such as: the world class commissioning assurance regime; *Commissioning Skills for the NHS*; the Principles and Rules for Collaboration and Competition; Guidance on the NHS Standard Contract[s]; the NHS Operating Framework for 2010/11; and NHS Standard Contracts. Combined, these create significant pressure for organisations to leave a clear audit trail of policies used, decisions made and processes used to arrive at decisions at every stage of procurement. PCTs must seek SHA approval for 'any decisions it identifies as potentially contentious' and for 'derogations from the standard three-year contract length'; and 'in all procurement the contract awarded must be the appropriate NHS Standard Contract, or appropriate Primary Care Contract'. These contracts typically run to 130-160 pages[2] and, in our experience, often encourage unnecessarily adversarial relationships between PCTs and providers.

Annex B

Different strategies for procurement and contract management

Taking a broad view, there are essentially two approaches to procurement across industry; what might be called the 'Japanese' approach and the 'adversarial' approach. These are described in summary form in Figure 2.

Figure 2:
Approaches to contracting and tendering

'Adversarial' Approach	'Japanese' Approach
<ul><li>Lack of trust;</li><li>'Squeeze suppliers bloodless';</li><li>Go for the best deal on cost;</li><li>No loyalty given or expected;</li><li>Mistakes of suppliers instantaneously punished;</li><li>Inflexible, bureaucratic and prescriptive contracting.</li></ul>	<ul><li>Collaboration with suppliers;</li><li>Building long-term relationships;</li><li>Encourage innovation: suppliers expected to invest in continuous improvement;</li><li>Loyalty valued. Suppliers rarely changed, although horizon constantly scanned for other solutions;</li><li>Mistakes sorted out collaboratively;</li><li>Flexible and informal contracting.</li></ul>
Consequences	**Consequences**
<ul><li>Suppliers in constant fear of losing contracts, therefore not prepared to invest in future;</li><li>Long, complex, inflexible supply agreements;</li><li>Tendering process expensive and time consuming.</li></ul>	<ul><li>Security from good performance encourages innovation;</li><li>Suppliers value reputation;</li><li>Better deals result;</li><li>Contracts are flexible and short in length covering the basics;</li><li>Costs of tendering are dramatically reduced.</li></ul>
Approach (generally) no longer used, with big improvements in the result.	*Approach continues today.*

The 'Japanese' approach is based on trust, and the expectation of a mutually beneficial long-term relationship of give-and-take; the 'adversarial' approach is based on mistrust, lengthy written contracts and the expectation that relationships will be adversarial as both purchaser and supplier try to outdo each other. In both models, suppliers accept that purchasers will horizon-scan for better deals on quality and cost, and most likely contract with a number of different suppliers to spur competition. However, in the Japanese model, although the 'threat' of exit always exists, it is recognised that changing suppliers is expensive; priority is given to flexibility and working with existing suppliers in order to improve on innovation elsewhere. In the adversarial model, business tends to be instantaneously switched.

The crucial point is that whereas the adversarial approach may score short-term gains, it is unlikely to be as successful in the long-run, because there is both no security to support innovation and the rigidity of contracts tends to prohibit it. Ford learnt this in the 1980s. It used to be the archetype 'adversarial' contractor, but abandoned this approach in light of the superior performance of Japanese car manufacturers.[1] In essence, Ford came to recognise, in the words of the economist John Kay, that 'in most commercial situations, it is impossible to specify all the contingencies that might arise. The formal contract is necessarily incomplete. Enforcement by reference to the explicit terms of the contract is therefore uncertain, expensive and largely irrelevant. The effective mechanism of enforcement is the need of the parties to go on doing business with each other'.[2] Contracts were reduced from volumes, to a few pages. In the intrinsically uncertain world of health care,[i] the Japanese approach is likely to be even more important.

---

[i] The evidence base about 'what works' in medicine is surprisingly slim. In fact, according to the *BMJ Clinical Evidence Handbook*, over 45 per cent of the medical activity commonly carried out in health systems lacks an evidence-base, and only 13 per cent is *proven* to be beneficial. This is not to say much of it is not clinically effective, but that it needs to be explored. Even less prevalent is evidence of cost-effectiveness (*BMJ Clinical Evidence Handbook*, London: BMJ Publishing, 2007; cited in: Maynard, A., *Payment for Performance (P4P): International experience and a cautionary proposal for Estonia*, Copenhagen: WHO Europe, 2008).

Annex C

The NHS in England:
The operating framework for 2008/9 – Principles and rules for co-operation and competition

These principles later formed the terms of reference for the Cooperation and Competition Panel (CCP), formed in 2009 to 'investigate and advise the DH and Monitor on potential breaches', relating to conduct, mergers, procurement and advertising.[1]

1. Commissioners should commission services from the providers who are best placed to deliver on the needs of their patients and population;

2. Providers and commissioners must cooperate to ensure that the patient experience is of a seamless health service, regardless of organisational boundaries, and to ensure service continuity and sustainability;

3. Commissioning and procurement should be transparent and non-discriminatory;

4. Commissioners and providers should foster patient choice and ensure that patients have accurate and reliable information to exercise more choice and control over their healthcare;

5. Appropriate promotional activity is encouraged as long as it remains consistent with patients' best interests and the brand and reputation of the NHS;

6. Providers must not discriminate against patients and must promote equality;

7. Payment regimes must be transparent and fair;

8. Financial intervention in the system must be transparent and fair;

9. Mergers, acquisitions, de-mergers and joint ventures are acceptable and permissible when they are demonstrated to be in patients' and taxpayers' best interests and there remains sufficient choice and

competition to ensure high quality standards of care and value for money;

10. Vertical integration is permissible when demonstrated to be in patients' and taxpayers' best interests and protects the primacy of the GP gatekeeper function; and there remains sufficient choice and competition to ensure high quality standards of care and value for money.

Notes

Summary

[1] Department of Health, *Operating Framework for 2008/9,* Annex D: Principles and Rules for Cooperation and Competition, London: TSO, 2007.

1: Introduction

[1] Appleby, J., Crawford, R. and Emmerson, C., *How Cold Will It Be? Prospects for NHS funding 2011-2017,* London: The King's Fund/IFS, 2009.

[2] Department of Health, *Departmental Reports (various),* London: TSO, 2010. http://www.dh.gov.uk/en/Publicationsandstatistics/Publications/PublicationsPolicyAndGuidance/DH_100667 (real terms calculations by authors, using HM Treasury GDP Deflator).

[3] Office for National Statistics (ONS), *Change in Healthcare Productivity, 1995 to 2008: News Release,* Newport: ONS, 24 March 2010, available at: http://www.statistics.gov.uk/pdfdir/health0310.pdf

[4] Department of Health, *Mortality Target Monitoring,* October 2009, http://www.dh.gov.uk/en/Publicationsandstatistics/Publications/PublicationsStatistics/DH_106776

[5] Berrino F. *et al.,* 'Survival for eight major cancers and all cancers combined for European adults diagnosed in 1995–99: results of the EUROCARE-4 study', *The Lancet Oncology,* 2007: 8(9); 773-783; Health at a Glance 2009, OECD, 8 December 2009.

[6] Klein, R., *The New Politics of the NHS: From Creation to Reinvention,* 5th edn, Oxford: Radcliffe, 2006.

[7] Brereton, L. and Vasoodaven, V., *The impact of the NHS market: an overview of the literature,* London: Civitas, 2010.

2: Background

[1] Brereton, L., and Vasoodaven, V., *The impact of the NHS market: an overview of the literature,* London: Civitas, 2010.

[2] Vickers, J., and Yarrow, G., *Privatization: An Economic Analysis,* Cambridge, Mass: MIT Press, 1988.

[3] Office of Fair Trading, *Productivity and Competition: An OFT perspective on the productivity debate,* London: OFT, 2007.

4   Office of Fair Trading, *Choice and Competition in Public Services: A guide for policy makers, A report prepared for the OFT by Frontier Economics*, London: OFT, 2010, p. 20.

5   Kay, J., *The Truth About Markets,* London: Penguin, 2004; Kay, J., 'The Failure of Market Failure', *Prospect,* Issue 137, August 2007 (specific to public services).

6   Kay, *The Truth About Markets*; Kay, 'The Failure of Market Failure', *Prospect,* Issue 137.

7   Office of Fair Trading, *Productivity and Competition: An OFT perspective on the productivity debate,* p. 12.

8   Office of Fair Trading, *Government in Markets: Why competition matters — a guide for policymakers,* London: OFT, 2009, Ch. 3.

9   Grace, C., Fletcher, K., Martin, S. and Bottrill, I., *Making and Managing Markets: Contestability, competition and improvement in local government, final report to the Audit Commission,* London: Audit Commission, November 2007.

10 Office of Fair Trading, *Productivity and Competition: An OFT perspective on the productivity debate.*

11 Cooper, Z. and Le Grand, J., 'Choice, competition and the left', *Eurohealth,* 13:4, 2008.

12 Aghion, P., Blundell, P., Griffith, R., Howitt, P, and Prantl, S., 'The Effect of Entry on Incumbent Innovation and Productivity', *The Review of Economics and Statistics,* 2009, Vol. 91.

13 Arrow, K.J., 'Uncertainty and the welfare economics of health care', *American Economic Review,* 1963, Vol. 53, No. 5, pp. 941–73. See also: Gubb, J., and Meller-Herbert, O., *Markets in Health Care: the theory behind the policy,* London: Civitas, 2009.

14 Enthoven, A., *In Pursuit of an Improving National Health Service,* London: The Nuffield Trust, 1999, ch. 4; Office of Fair Trading, *Choice and Competition in Public Services: A guide for policy makers* A report prepared for the OFT by Frontier Economics, London: OFT, 2010.

15 Bevan, G. and van de Ven, W.P.M.M., 'Choice of providers and mutual healthcare purchasers: can the English National Health Service learn from the Dutch reforms?', *Health Economics, Policy and Law,* available on Cambridge Journals Online (CJO), 18 May 2010, doi:10.1017/S1744133110000071; Ferlie, E. and Shortell, S., 'Improving The Quality of Health Care in the UK and USA – A Framework for Change', *Milbank Quarterly,* 2001, 79(2): 281-315.

16 Department of Health, *Working for Patients*, Cm 555, London: HMSO, 1989.

17 Bevan, G. and Hood, C., 'Have targets improved performance in the English NHS?', *BMJ*, 2006, 332:419-22.

18 Stevens, S., 'Reform strategies for the English NHS', *Health Affairs*, 2004, Vol. 23, No. 3, pp. 41–44.

19 Department of Health, *Delivering the NHS Plan: next steps on investment, next steps on reform*, Cm 5503, London: HSMO, 2002.

20 Department of Health, *World Class Commissioning: Practice-based commissioning in action, a guide for GPs*, London: TSO, 2009.

21 Ernst & Young LLP, *Understanding health care markets: A PCT guide to market analysis and market management*, London: Ernst & Young, 2009.

22 Department of Health, *Delivering the NHS Plan: Next steps on investment, next steps on reform*.

23 Department of Health, *Health Reform in England: Update and next steps*, London: TSO, 2005.

24 Dixon, A., *et al.*, *Patient Choice: How patients choose and how providers respond*, London: The King's Fund, 2010, Introduction.

25 Blair, T., *We must not waste this precious period of power*, speech given at South Camden Community College, 23 January 2003, cited in: Appleby, J., Harrison, A. and Devlin, N., *What is the Real Cost of More Patient Choice?*, London: The King's Fund, 2003, available at: www.kingsfund.org.uk/publications/what_is_the_real.html

26 Cooper, Z. and Le Grand, J., 'Choice, competition and the left', *Eurohealth*, 13:4, 2008.

27 Blair, T., speech on public services delivered at Guys and St Thomas' Hospital London, 23 June 2004, available at http://news.bbc.co.uk/1/hi/uk_politics/3833345.stm

28 Department of Health, *Departmental Reports (various)*, London: TSO, 2010. http://www.dh.gov.uk/en/Publicationsandstatistics/Publications/PublicationsPolicyAndGuidance/DH_100667 (real terms calculations by authors, using HM Treasury GDP Deflator).

29 Appleby, J., Crawford, R. and Emmerson, C., *How Cold Will It Be? Prospects for NHS funding 2011-2017*, London: The King's Fund/IFS, 2009.

30 Phelps, M., *Total Public Service Output and Productivity*, UK Centre for the Measurement of Government Activity, London: ONS (revised version published on 14 August 2009).

31 Propper, C., 'Competition and Choice', presentation to the Nuffield Trust Health Strategy Summit, March 2009, available at: http://www.nuffieldtrust.org.uk/downloads/detail.aspx?id=514 (accessed 1 July 2010).

32 Gaynor, M., *What do we Know about Competition and Quality in Health Care Markets?*, Cambridge, Mass: NBER, 2006, Working Paper 12301.

33 Propper, C., Wilson, D. and Burgess, S., 'Extending choice in English health care: the implications of the economic evidence', *Journal of Social Policy*, 2006, Vol. 35, No. 4, pp. 537–57.

34 Gaynor, M., Moreno-Serra, R. and Propper, C., *Death by Market Power: Reform, competition and patient outcomes in the National Health Service*, Cambridge, Mass: NBER, 2010, Working Paper No. 16164; Cooper, Z.N., McGuire, A., Jones, S. and Le Grand, J., 'Equity, waiting times, and NHS reforms: retrospective study', *BMJ*, 3 September 2009, 339: b3264; Cooper, Z., Gibbons, S., Jones, S. and McGuire, A., *Does Hospital Competition Save Lives? Evidence From The English NHS Patient Choice Reforms*, LSE Working Paper No. 16/2010, 2010; Bloom, N., Propper, C., Seiler, S. and Van Reenen, J., *The Impact of Competition on Management Quality: Evidence from public hospitals*, CEP Discussion Paper, May 2010, No. 983; Cooper, Z., Gibbons, S., Jones, S. and McGuire, A., *Does Hospital Competition Improve Efficiency? An Analysis of the Recent Market-Based Reforms to the English NHS*, London: Centre for Economic Performance, June 2010, CEPDP0988.

35 Brereton, L., and Vasoodaven, V., *The impact of the NHS market: an overview of the literature*, London: Civitas, 2010.

36 Lawson, N., *Machines, Markets and Morals: The new politics of a democratic NHS*, London: Compass, 2008.

37 See: http://www.lookafterournhs.org.uk/

3: Methodology

1 Brereton, L. and Vasoodaven, V., *The impact of the NHS market: an overview of the literature*, London: Civitas, 2010.

2 Gubb, J., and Meller-Herbert, O., *Markets in health care: the theory behind the policy*, London: Civitas, 2009.

3   Office of Fair Trading, *Productivity and Competition: An OFT perspective on the productivity debate*, London: OFT, 2007.

4   Marshall, M., 'Sampling for qualitative research', *Family Practice* 1996; 13: 522-525.

4: Core Findings

1   Dixon, A., *et al.*, *Patient Choice: How patients choose and how providers respond*, London: The King's Fund, 2010.

5: Is the Concept of a Market in the NHS Flawed?

1   Zwarenstein, M., Goldman, J. and Reeves, S., 'Interprofessional collaboration: effects of practice-based interventions on professional practice and healthcare outcomes', *Cochrane Database of Systematic Reviews* 2009, Issue 3, Art. No.: CD000072; Barbieri, A., Vanhaecht, K. *et al.*, 'Effects of clinical pathways in the joint replacement: a meta-analysis, *BMC Medicine*, 1 July 2009, 7:32.

2   Department of Health, *Operating Framework for 2008/9*, Annex D: Principles and Rules for Cooperation and Competition, London: TSO, 2007.

3   Burnham, A., 'NHS as preferred provider', Dear Colleague Letter, London: Department of Health, 13 October 2009, Gateway Reference Number: 12774.

4   Propper, C., Sutton, M., Whitnall, C. and Windmeijer, F., 'Did "targets and terror" reduce waiting times in England for hospital care?', *The B.E. Journal of Economic Analysis & Policy*, 2008, Vol. 8, Iss. 2 (Contributions), Article 5.

5   Shekelle, P. G., Lim, Y., Mattke, S. and Damberg, C., *Does Public Release of Performance Results Improve Quality of Care? A systematic review*, London: Health Foundation, 2008.

6   Office of Fair Trading, *Choice and Competition in Public Services: A guide for policy makers*; A report prepared for the OFT by Frontier Economics, London: OFT, 2010.

7   Cooper, Z.N., McGuire, A., Jones, S. and Le Grand, J., 'Equity, waiting times, and NHS reforms: retrospective study', *BMJ*, 3 September 2009, 339: b3264; Cooper, Z., Gibbons, S., Jones, S. and McGuire, A., *Does Hospital Competition Save Lives? Evidence From The English NHS Patient Choice Reforms*, London: LSE, 2010 Working Paper, No. 16/2010; Bloom, N., Propper, C., Seiler, S. and Van Reenen, J., *The Impact of Competition on Management Quality: Evidence from public hospitals*, CEP Discussion Paper, May 2010, No. 983; Cooper, Z., Gibbons, S., Jones, S., McGuire, A., *Does Hospital Competition Improve Efficiency? An analysis of the*

recent market-based reforms to the English NHS, London: Centre for Economic Performance, June 2010, CEPDP0988.

6: Is the Market Being Distorted and Stifled?

[1] Office of Fair Trading, *Choice and Competition in Public Services: A guide for policy makers*, London: OFT, 2010.

[2] Office of Fair Trading, *Choice and Competition in Public Services*.

[3] Sussex, J., *How Fair? Competition between independent and NHS providers to supply non-emergency hospital care to NHS patients in England*, London: Office of Health Economics, 2009.

[4] Enthoven, A., *In Pursuit of an Improving National Health Service*, London: The Nuffield Trust, 1999.

[5] Dixon, J., Chantler, C. and Billings, J., *Competition on Outcomes and Physician Leadership are not Enough to Reform Health Care*, JAMA, 2007;298:1445-1447; Department of Health, *The NHS Operating Framework for England for 2010/11*, London: TSO, 2009.

[6] Gaynor, M., *What do we Know about Competition and Quality in Health Care Markets?*, Cambridge, MA: National Bureau of Economic Research, 2006.

[7] Le Grand, J., Mays, N. and Mulligan, J. (eds), *Learning from the NHS Internal Market*, London: The King's Fund, 1998.

[8] Department of Health, *PCT Procurement Guide for Health Services*, London: TSO, 2010.

[9] Brereton, L. and Vasoodaven, V., *The Impact of the NHS Market: An overview of the literature*, London: Civitas, 2010; Harvey, S., Liddell, A., McMahon, L., *Windmill 2009: NHS response to the financial storm*, London: The King's Fund, 2009.

[10] Department of Health, *ISTC Market Sustainability Analysis*, February 2005.

7: What Should be Done?

[1] Appleby, J., Crawford, R. and Emmerson, C., *How cold will it be? Prospects for NHS funding 2011-2017*, London: The King's Fund/IFS, 2009.

[2] Office of Fair Trading, *Productivity and Competition: An OFT perspective on the productivity debate*, London: OFT, 2007.

[3] Dixon, A. *et al.*, *Patient Choice: How patients choose and how providers respond*, London: The King's Fund, 2010.

4   Department of Health, *ISTC Market Sustainability Analysis*, February 2005.

5   Department of Health, *Operating Framework for 2008/9,* Annex D: Principles and Rules for Cooperation and Competition, London: TSO, 2007.

Annex A

1   Department of Health, *PCT Procurement Guide for Health Services*, London: TSO, 2010.

2   Department of Health, Guidance on the NHS Standard Contract for Acute Services 2010/11, London: TSO, 2010.

Annex B

1   Charman, K., 'The NHS in the simulator: What the NHS can learn from Ford in the 1980s', *BMJ*, 2010, 340:c297.

2   Kay, J., 'Think before you tear up an unwritten contract', *The Financial Times*, 16 March 2010.

Annex C

1   http://www.ccpanel.org.uk/about-the-ccp/index.html

Further Civitas publications:*

Putting Patients Last: How the NHS keeps the ten commandments of business failure
Peter Davies and James Gubb, July 2009
Cover Price: £7.50
Special online price: £2
ISBN: 978-1-906837-09-9

Quite like heaven? Options for the NHS in a consumer age
Nick Seddon, November 2007
Cover price: £12
Special online price: £1
ISBN: 978-1-903386-63-7

A New Inquisition: Religious persecution in Britain today
Jon Gower Davies, July 2010
Cover price: £6
Special online price: £4
ISBN: 978-1-906837-15-0

Social Mobility Myths
Peter Saunders, June 2010
Cover price: £8
Special online price: £5
ISBN: 978-1-906837-14-3

Prosperity with Principles: Some policies for economic growth
David G. Green, April 2010
Cover price: £6
Special online price: £4
ISBN: 978-1906837-13-6

Postage & packing: £2.75 per book, £1.50 for each subsequent book.

To purchase publications, or to order a full catalogue, please contact:

Book Sales, Civitas, 55 Tufton Street, London, SW1P 3QL
Tel: 020 7799 6677
Fax: 020 7799 6688
Email: books@civitas.org.uk
Web: http://www.civitas.org.uk/shop/

Note: These prices are correct at the time of publication.